271
.T9
1997

Arthur G. Tweet, Ph.D.
Karol Gavin-Marciano

# The Guide to

# Benchmarking
# in Healthcare

Practical
Lessons
From
the
Field

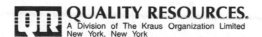 **QUALITY RESOURCES.**
A Division of The Kraus Organization Limited
New York, New York

Most Quality Resources books are available at quantity discounts when purchased in bulk. For more information contact:

Special Sales Department
Quality Resources
A Division of the Kraus Organization Limited
902 Broadway                                       800-247-8519
New York, New York 10010                 212-979-8600
www.qualityresources.com            E-mail: info@qualityresources.com

Printed in the United States of America

02 01 00 99 98        10 9 8 7 6 5 4 3 2 1
                                ∞
The paper used in this publication meets the minimum requirements of American National Standard for Information Sciences—Permanence of Paper for Printed Library Materials, ANSI Z39.48-1984.

ISBN 0-527-76337-3

**Library of Congress Cataloging-in-Publication Data**

Tweet, Arthur G.
        The guide to benchmarking in healthcare : practical lessons from the field / Arthur G. Tweet, Karol Gavin-Marciano.
                p.        cm.
        Includes bibliographical references and index..
        ISBN 0-527-76337-3 (alk. paper)
        1. Health services administration.  2. Benchmarking (management) I. Gavin-Marciano, Karol.  II. Title.
RA971.T9     1997
362.1'068—dc21                                                                97-34887
                                                                                        CIP

# Contents

# Acknowledgments

The authors wish to acknowledge help from a number of people in the preparation of the case studies in this book. We thank Jeanne Dent, R.N., Associate Quality Officer (Ret.), Strong Memorial Hospital, who provided help on the blood bank case study, and much general encouragement on the entire project. We are grateful to Curtis Benesch, M.D., Assistant Professor of Neurology, the university of Rochester Medical School, for sharing his experiences and for his helpful comments on the stroke therapy case. We thank Rita L. Radcliffe, M.D. MBA, Vice-President for Medical Affairs and Corporate Medical Director, Health Services Medical Corporation of Central NY, Inc., for consultation and critique of the HMO case study. We thank Sandy Griffin-Roth of the Canadaigua, NY VAMC for her helpful comments on the computer systems change-over case study.

For help on the chapter concerning the Internet it is a pleasure to acknowledge the very helpful support of Patricia Letendre, Assistant Professor, Division of Medical Laboratory Science, University of Alberta. We also acknowledge very useful conversations with Anne T. and Craig F. Knoche, Principals, Summit Performance Group, Inc., as well as with Neil Blumberg, M.D., Professor of Pathology and Laboratory Medicine at the University of Rochester School of Medicine and Dentistry.

For all their support, encouragement, and forebearance, we thank with deepest gratitude our respective spouses, Thea S. Tweet and Joseph P. Marciano.

Finally, for a book of this sort, which attempts to distill the experiences of scores of benchmarking teams over a period of nearly 20 years, it is impossible to give proper credit to all the people who contributed to its content. Any helpful insights that this book may contain were developed through observing their efforts. We hope that the team members will understand and forgive our inability to acknowledge them individually.

Rochester, New York

September 1997

# Introduction

Benchmarking is the process of identifying best practices, and adopting or adapting them for your own use. It is a highly effective tool for discovering and implementing the proper approach for getting work done.

Benchmarking is widely practiced in the world of business. It is used to improve how companies carry out activities as different as manufacturing, new product development, finance, marketing, sales, and field service.

In the world of healthcare, one of the essential functions of benchmarking — identification of best practice — is already being done in many of the clinical disciplines. Practice, Parameters, Critical Pathways, and Case Management protocols all concern the identification of best practices. Organizations such as the College of American Pathologists, with its Q-Probes Benchmarking Program, and the American Academy of Pediatrics, with its ACQIP program, focus on improving the quality of their particular medical specialties. The Institute for Healthcare Improvement's Quality Management Network addresses healthcare best practice delivery from the institutional point of view.

Unfortunately, simply *identifying* the best practices does not necessarily lead automatically to their *use*. All too often, clinicians find little sympathy for their ideas from support groups and the people in administrative posts. Conversely, administrators often find it difficult or impossible to convince doctors, nurses, and allied health professionals of the benefits of needed changes identified by the administrative staff. As a consequence, little or nothing is done to put the best practices to use.

This is where benchmarking has its greatest value. It provides the framework for both *finding better ways* to provide healthcare and *building consensus for using them*.

We have tried to make this benchmarking book accessible for very busy people. Everyone who is involved in, or will be affected by, a benchmarking project will benefit from reading this book. However, some sections are more applicable than others to the specific roles in the benchmarking process. Accordingly, the book is structured to easily find and read the sections that describe the parts of the process immediately relevant to what you are trying to do at the moment.

For example, if you are:

- A *leader in the medical staff*, you are probably already doing many of the most important steps in benchmarking, some perhaps *via* the Internet. By learning how to build support for your findings in your home environment, your efforts will prove more effective. Read Chapter 6, The Ischemic Stroke Case Study, first.

- A *department head*, you may be called upon to supervise a benchmarking project. You will do a better job if you learn the most effective ways to ensure the project's success. Read Chapter 5, The Blood Bank Performance Improvement Case Study, first.

- A *person in top management*, one of your main responsibilities is to bring fresh ideas into your organization. Learn how to ensure that these new ideas directly address your key strategic goals and gain enthusiastic support within the organization. Read Chapter 7, The Cranbrook Health Systems Modernization Crisis Case Study, first.

- A *chief information officer*, you know there is more to bringing new computer systems on-line than simply installing new hardware and software. Learn what benchmarking can do to help smooth the transition within your user community. Read Chapter 8, the St. Luke's Hospital Information System Changeover Case Study, first.

- A *first-line supervisor*, you may be called upon to participate in a benchmarking project, either as a team member or an expert consultant. Learn what benchmarking is about to ensure that the project makes best use of available expertise. Read Chapter 5, The Blood Bank Performance Improvement Case Study, first.

Each case study includes things that go well and things that don't, just as in the real world. For the same reason, the expository material includes candid discussions of how human nature and other problems can influence the benchmarking process. For example, considerable space in the book is devoted to the peculiarities of human behavior in situations involving risk, job threat, and other emotionally loaded issues. However, as a timesaver, we have eschewed histrionic dramatization in almost all instances except the information case study, in which it was needed to highlight a point.

In the interest of making benchmarking more accessible to the busy professional, we have also tried to avoid using the jargon of the quality movement. Little knowledge of this terminology is needed to read the book—or do benchmarking. (The first two major benchmarking projects done in the United States by Xerox were completed even before the term *benchmarking* was coined!) We have treated the general descriptions of the benchmarking process in terms familiar to all healthcare workers, and have set the case studies in familiar healthcare environments.

Also, in deference to the readers' busy schedules, we have largely dispensed with theoretical and historical background references and discussion. This book is more a how-to manual than a treatise.

As a practical matter, we recognize that the full participation of medical staff members in benchmarking projects is virtually impossible. (Indeed, these natural intellectual leaders in the organization may be seen as critics rather than as participants in organized attempts to change and improve many of the work processes of healthcare.) In recognition of this fact, we have shown in two of the case studies, the blood bank case and the stroke treatment case, how alternative roles for the medical staff can be found that involve a minimum investment of their time, but do make good use of their talents.

## STRUCTURE OF THIS BOOK

The book is broken into three major parts: Principles and Process, Case Studies, and Special Topics, followed by a set of tutorial Appendixes and a list of references.

*Part I: Principles and Process.* This part describes the four phases and 12 individual steps of a benchmarking project in general language. It serves as a quick reference guide with checklists for what needs to be done in a benchmarking project, and at what stage. To make it easier to keep track of where you are in the process, we will use the process road-map in Figure 1. Also, whenever a new term with a specialized meaning in benchmarking is introduced, it will be boldface at first use.

**Figure 1. Road-map.**

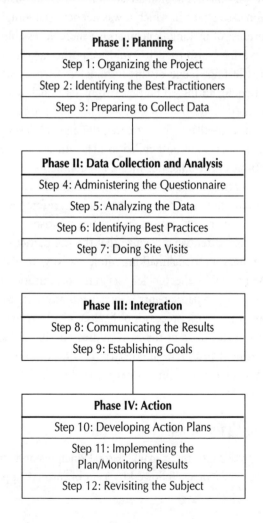

# Introduction

Throughout Part I, *icons* of the road-map marked with shading will appear in the margins to indicate what part of the process is being discussed in the text. For example, the icon in the margin of this paragraph identifies Step 3 of Phase I as its subject.

In Part I, where possible, we have emphasized the use of methods for *identification* of best practices that are already familiar to healthcare providers. These are ways of using existing networks of formal and informal contacts to obtain and disseminate information. They are well adapted to the culture of healthcare providers, making it easier to get started on a benchmarking effort.

However, because the ultimate goal of benchmarking is to *use the best identifiable practices*, we will emphasize ways to extend and supplement already familiar management methods to make them more effective in achieving this ultimate goal.

*Part II: Case Studies.* The case studies are detailed descriptions of four different fictitious benchmarking projects. Each study is presented from the perspective of one of four main categories of players:

- Benchmarking team leader and team members
- Project sponsor (the project's immediate customer)
- Top management
- Members of the affected workforce

It is not necessary to read all four case studies to understand the benchmarking process from any one of these perspectives. However, in order to appreciate some of the subtleties of the interactions among participants, we recommend that you do so. This is particularly true for benchmarking team leaders, quality officers, and others in leadership positions in organizations that plan to do benchmarking.

Each case study is told in a short-story format, with the key project documents and process descriptions woven into the text and set off with outline boxes. As in Part I, the *icons* in the margins provide at-a-glance ties to the benchmarking phase being portrayed as the story unfolds.

| PHASE I PLANNING |
|---|
| Step 1: Organizing the Project |
| Step 2: Identifying Best Practitioners |
| Step 3: Preparing to Collect Data |

By concentrating on the actions of a particular category of player, and simply sketching the activities of the other role categories, it has been possible to keep the case studies short. For example, the case study from the project team perspective includes a complete set of minutes from the team meetings. The case study from the sponsoring department head's perspective, however, does not even mention such team-related documentation, focusing instead on the sponsor's own actions on behalf of the team.

Also in the interest of brevity, we have largely avoided the strictly technical aspects of the subject matter. For example, in the case study on the Ischemic Stroke Initiative in Part II, the benchmarking project concerns how to make the new treatment work, but steers clear of the medical details associated with the use of tissue plasminogen activator.

*Part III: Special Topics.* Two additional chapters address topics of special interest and importance:

- Use of the Internet as a tool in each of the phases of benchmarking.
- The benchmarking of cost and how it could be used in preparing for capitation.

Appendixes. — Three appendixes can be found at the end of the book detailing how-to discussions of team building, the preparation of questionnaires, and action planning in Phase IV, all of which are vital to the success of a benchmarking project.

# Part I

# Principles and Process

## OVERVIEW

Benchmarking is a management tool. It should be used

- when you want to find out where your services rank in the community of your peers and how much they might be improved,

                    and

- when you know *what* you want to do, but are not sure *how to do it*, whether it be the improvement of an existing product or service or the introduction of one that is new to your organization.

It is therefore most useful for *setting goals* for the future course of an organization and for *doing* the things necessary to begin achieving those goals.

## SETTING GOALS

Benchmarking is a window on the world that makes available a steady stream of new ideas from the outside, enabling constructive dialogue with other healthcare organizations with similar problems and interests. It also facilitates the study of best practices of organizations from other sectors of the economy that may be relevant to the needs of healthcare.

## Doing

Benchmarking is a framework for leadership in initiating action within an organization based on institutional priorities, helping to build consensus at all organizational levels about key measures of success. It is a valuable tool for transferring ownership of performance goals to the people who will be accountable for achieving them — both for bringing new services into the institution and for improving existing work processes.

# THE 12-STEP BENCHMARKING PROCESS

Benchmarking is a process that can be broken down into four phases: Planning, Data Collection and Analysis, Integration, and Action. The phases are divided into 12 steps, each of which comprises a number of activities.

Figure 1. The 12-step benchmarking process.

### Phase I – Planning

Step 1: Organizing the Project
- Selecting the subject
- Selecting the team leader
- Recruiting the team
- Building the team
- Developing a team charter

Step 2: Identifying the Best Practitioners
- Positioning the project
- Seeking benchmarking partner sources

Step 3: Preparing to Collect Data
- Flow-charting the process
- Identifying requirements for success for the project
- Using information sources
- Developing questionnaires
- Recruiting benchmarking partners
- Answering your own questionnaires

**Phase II – Data Collection and Analysis**

Step 4: Administering the Questionnaire
- – Full-scale questionnaires
- – Short-form questionnaires

Step 5: Analyzing the Data
- – Compiling the responses
- – Identifying the benchmarks and gap profile
- – Reviewing the findings

Step 6: Identifying Best Practices
- – Understanding best practices
- – Identifying opportunities
- – Making gap projections
- – Preparing draft recommendations

Step 7: Doing Site Visits
- – Picking a site visit scenario
- – Site visit protocol
- – Updating findings and draft recommendations

**Phase III – Integration**

Step 8: Communicating the Results
- – Strategy and process
- – Content

Step 9: Establishing Goals
- – Completing ownership transfer

**Phase IV – Action**

Step 10: Developing Action Plans
- – Planning
- – Communication

Step 11: Implementing the Plan/Monitoring Results

Step 12: Revisiting the Subject

---

Following are some comments about the 12-step process:

- There is nothing really new in this process. The activities in all of the phases are familiar to most managers. The exceptional strength of the process lies in the fact that it *is* a process: the phases are carried out together and in sequence. Taken individually, they lack this power. For example, when planning is done in isolation, for its own sake, the output is a report that usually gathers dust in credenzas and libraries. Similarly, data collection alone produces columns of figures that no one acts upon, and analysis done without a purpose is sterile.

- The phases in the process should be done in sequence, with all the work in each phase completed before going on to the next phase.

- It is very important at the end of each phase to check to see that all the work done to date produces a self-consistent picture. For example, in the Ischemic Stroke Initiative case in Chapter 6, the benchmarking team began looking at subjects outside the scope of their charter — their work was not *self-consistent*. Everything — the objective, the team composition, the team work plan, the questionnaire, etc. — must go together.

- It is by no means essential, however, to follow the individual steps within a phase in strict sequence, particularly in Phase I. It is quite possible in Phase I that a benchmarking team will wish to go quickly through all of Steps 1, 2, and 3 before completing the work in Step 1: Organizing the Project. For example, it is frequently the case that in preparing to collect the data in Step 3, a benchmarking team will gain deeper insight into the true nature of their subject, and make appropriate adjustments to what they did in Step 1 so as to restore *self-consistency*.

- It is not essential that an organization be practicing Total Quality Management/Continuous Quality Improvement (TQM/CQI) in order to carry out a benchmarking project. However, the basic tenets of benchmarking are very closely allied with those of TQM/CQI, and a few key ideas and terms from TQM/CQI must be understood by all stakeholders in a benchmarking project if the process is to go smoothly:

- The elemental sequence in work is that **inputs** are converted into **outputs** by means of work processes in a work environment.

- A **quality output** is one that has the characteristics it is supposed to have — specifically, the characteristics promised to the recipient (usually called **"the customer"**).

- A **quality process** is one that performs the way it is supposed to, producing a quality output.

- In most situations, bad outputs are produced by faulty processes, not faulty people.

- The way to improve an output is to improve the process that produces it. This might be called the **Golden Rule of TQM/CQI.**

- One important mark of an improved process is that there is reduced *variation* in the output.

- Only the people who do the work know how the work actually gets done. This is the compelling reason for practicing what is usually called **employee involvement.**

# ROLES AND RESPONSIBILITIES

We have seen that benchmarking is a tool used for setting new goals and initiating the actions needed to achieve these goals. It can be used in any part of an organization, or at any level. However, benchmarking is intended to produce changes to the operating plan and usually to the budget, which are the province of management. Therefore, its use must have concurrence and support at appropriately high levels of management.

In the following description of roles and responsibilities, it is assumed that the benchmarking project will be overseen by the top management of the organization. This is by no means always the case, but will be if the subject addresses a major new service initiated by top management or cuts across major organizational lines. The Ischemic Stroke Initiative in Chapter 6 is an example of a major new service. The blood bank case in Chapter 5 depicts strong interactions among many departments in the hospital. In the latter instance, even though the project was initiated fairly far down in the organization, its oversight became a top management concern.

In situations where the benchmarking project objective does not involve the top levels in the organization, the roles of the executive committee and the sponsor may be combined. A department director, for example, may charter a benchmarking team for which he or she is the only customer.

## ROLE OF THE EXECUTIVE COMMITTEE

This committee is made up of the CEO and her/his direct reports: top management. Its role in benchmarking is to ensure that projects address high-priority subjects of strategic importance. Chapter 7 depicts the roles of a CEO and his executive committee. Specific actions are to:

- Require that the benchmarking project has a clear goal.

- Appoint a **sponsor**, preferably one who is a member of the executive committee. The sponsor represents the executive committee to the benchmarking team and is the project's **immediate customer**.

- Establish a policy that the work done on benchmarking projects is a major performance objective for team members, probably requiring reprioritization of other scheduled activities for team members.

- Require periodic reviews of team progress. For a large project, reviews may be carried out by a steering committee led by the team sponsor. Projects of a more modest size probably will not need such a structure, review by the team sponsor being sufficient.

- Require that the benchmarking project final report include actionable recommendations that are consistent with the institution's strategic plan.

- Ensure that recommendations that have been concurred are properly prioritized and incorporated in a timely fashion into the operating plan and budget.

## ROLE OF THE TEAM SPONSOR

The team sponsor has a dual role. He or she is the benchmarking team's immediate customer, but is also the project's "friend in court" who is able to smooth the way for the project. The sponsor is usually a person high in management, with enough recognition in all parts of the organization to carry out both of these functions effectively. Chapter 6 focuses on this role, which comprises the following responsibilities:

- Recruit a **team leader**.
- Support the team leader in recruiting benchmarking team members.
- Work closely with the team leader to establish a **team charter** and a team protocol or work process that ensures credibility of the project results. (The team charter is the project plan. It describes what will be done, why it will be done, how it will be done, who will do it, in what sequence, and according to what schedule the actions will occur.)
- Ensure the availability of adequate resources (e.g., consultation from functional experts, required data, etc.).
- Conduct periodic reviews of the project's progress.
- Inform the executive committee regularly of team progress.
- Ensure that team output recommendations will be acceptable to the executive committee, the customer group that the sponsor represents.

## ROLE OF THE TEAM LEADER

The team leader will be responsible for delivering a set of action recommendations (the key project output) to the sponsor, who is the benchmarking project's immediate customer. However, the team leader/sponsor relationship is by no means at arms-length, but much more like the vendor–customer partnerships that have proven so effective in industry worldwide. The team leader is usually a person with supervisory experience who has high credibility with the organization that will be most directly associated with the new or improved process. If the **process owner** (the supervisor who is accountable for the process) is well known to be objective and receptive to new ideas, she/he may be chosen as team leader. The team leader's responsibilities include:

- Recruit team members whose combined knowledge adequately covers all key aspects of the subject to be benchmarked.

- Provide the benchmarking team with all necessary information about relevant aspects of the strategic plan and the current operating plan.

- Be responsible for all aspects of team leadership and administration, including recruitment of a facilitator if necessary.

- Ensure that planning professionals (financial analysts, facilities planners, etc.) assist the team to state its findings and recommendations so as to make them actionable in the context of the next cycle of the operating (budgetary) plan.

# Chapter 1

# Phase I: Planning

*Phase I begins when an organization wishes to initiate a new service or to improve its current performance in some area, recognizing that a benchmarking project is needed. Phase I continues to the point where detailed information-gathering is begun to determine how other organizations have achieved superior results.*

Along the way you will answer a number of key questions:

What exactly will we benchmark and why?

Who will do the work?

What is the purpose of the **team charter**?

Who will be our **benchmarking partners**?

How will we know if the project is successful?

What information will we collect from our benchmarking partners?

How will we compare this information with information obtained from our own organization?

How will we obtain the needed information, both internally and externally?

At the conclusion of Phase I, the team will be ready to collect and analyze data.

| PHASE I
PLANNING |
| :---: |
| Step 1:
Organizing
the Project |
| Step 2:
Identifying Best
Practitioners |
| Step 3:
Preparing to
Collect Data |

# STEP 1: ORGANIZING THE PROJECT
## SELECTING THE SUBJECT

A successful benchmarking project begins with a specific functional **objective**, brought on either by a desire to innovate or by dissatisfaction with the *status quo*. If the objective is part of the overall corporate strategy, it should be selected by the executive committee. If it is a quality improvement objective at the departmental level, it should be selected by, or with concurrence of, the department head. Regardless of the subject or its scope, the process should always be roughly the same:

- State the objective as clearly as possible: "This is what I want to do (or do better)." For example,

  – An executive committee may decide it wants to start an organ transplant program.

  – A pathology laboratory head may want to reduce the cost of running the laboratory.

- Then ask "I wonder what an attainable goal is, and how I should go about achieving it?"

  – The executive committee may wonder whether its institution could become one of the top five liver transplant centers in North America, and what it should do to get there.

  – The laboratory head may wonder if the lab's total cost of operation might be reduced by 40%, and how that might be safely achieved.

While the overall *objective* should be carefully thought out and stated, too much precision in the statement of the benchmarking project **goal** is *un*desirable at this point. You may know where you want to go, but you probably don't yet know what to concentrate on in order to get there. For example, the laboratory director would not want to focus on reducing supplies cost at this stage, because this may not be the most important cost-reduction opportunity for the lab.

10

This important point is illustrated fully in the first case study in Part II, where a hospital blood bank supervisor has an *objective* — to improve the overall operation of her blood bank — but she doesn't know how to do it. From several aspects of the blood bank's operation, she selects Improving Blood Components Delivery as the general subject of her benchmarking project. Since she is not sure exactly what improvements are needed, she leaves that open-ended for the time being. By doing so, she gives the people on her benchmarking team, as well as others, the opportunity to contribute to her understanding of the problems she faces. If she had not kept the subject area general, she would have run the risk of asking her team to work on a problem of relatively minor importance.

| PHASE I PLANNING |
| --- |
| **Step 1:** Organizing the Project |
| **Step 2:** Identifying Best Practitioners |
| **Step 3:** Preparing to Collect Data |

Later, after the team leader and benchmarking team have been recruited and the blood bank supervisor has made the general project objective clear to them, the team is able to sharpen and refine the project goals as part of their job. In the Blood Bank example, the team arrived at very specific goals for the project: to benchmark the time and cost needed to deliver an order for blood components and to obtain detailed knowledge of the best delivery practices available for study.

## SELECTING THE TEAM LEADER

If the project is initiated by upper management, choosing the leader of a benchmarking team is part of the sponsor's job. If the project is initiated from lower in the organization, as in the Blood Bank case study, it may work the other way around, with the team leader finding a high-level sponsor. (See pages 7 and 8, for a description of the sponsor and team leader roles and how they interact.) Regardless of how it gets started, the sponsor and the team leader must form a close partnership, so the personal chemistry must be good. The sponsor attends to maintaining a supportive working environment, allowing the team to do its best work, while the team leader attends to the actual work of the team. The team leader must be able to function independently, with a minimum of day-to-day advice about what to do; otherwise, the sponsor will end up being the *de facto* team leader.

| PHASE I PLANNING |
| :---: |
| **Step 1:** Organizing the Project |
| **Step 2:** Identifying Best Practitioners |
| **Step 3:** Preparing to Collect Data |

Since the leader must lead in group situations, she or he should have had some previous supervisory experience. It is also important that the team leader be attuned to both formal and informal management mechanisms of the organization, and must not be dismayed by situations involving turf, status, and the like.

Both the risks and the rewards of team leadership must be understood by both team leader and team sponsor. The team leader's job should become one of the formal job objectives of the person in that role, with clearly defined performance measures tied to the overall organizational objective driving the benchmarking project.

There can be no hard and fast rules about the time commitment required for a team leader. Team size, technical and organizational complexity, availability of support staff, and time constraints all enter the equation. It is seldom the case, however, that a professionally competent, widely acquainted, and organizationally savvy manager will be willingly spared from his or her regular job on a more than half-time basis, and even that is ambitious. On the other hand, when the potential for influencing the future course of the institution's fortunes is considered, it is hard to imagine how anyone could object to freeing up the best-qualified person for the job. If a benchmarking project is important enough to be worth doing, it is important enough to be worth doing well, and that starts with getting the right person to run it. If that means that the project has to take a little longer for completion, this may be the only logical solution.

## RECRUITING THE TEAM

Team recruitment is a key responsibility shared by both the team leader and team sponsor. Executive and peer support for the project must be obtained at the outset. Once supervisory people understand the goals of a benchmarking project and the favorable results the organization as a whole and/or their own operation will enjoy, they will be more likely to support the project and agree to participation by their people.

Since the single biggest cost involved with a benchmarking project is the team members' time, *it is important not to minimize the*

12

*difficulties likely to be encountered in team recruiting.* Good benchmarking team members should have a broad knowledge of the work processes relevant to the general subject, the highest professional regard among their peers, should be good team players, and should be willing to participate in the project. Such people do not grow on trees, and must be courted.

The time commitment required of benchmarking team members will be determined by the size and complexity of the project and how urgently results are needed. The project may require only a few hours a week or up to half an employee's time. It should not be considered an "extra" to be done on "nights and weekends," although it is likely that some of the work will be done outside of regular hours.

In an effort to protect participants, team membership must be considered a formal job assignment included as one of the individual's performance objectives. It should be rated according to the organization's standard criteria (interpersonal skills, initiative, performance, etc.) at performance appraisal time by the team leader and the sponsor (or by the other team members in an organization with self-managing work groups).

The selection of the team roster requires a balance between a team where all the **stakeholders** — the groups whose own work will be affected by the results of the benchmarking project — are represented on the team, and one that is small enough to be able to function effectively. When all stakeholders are represented, communication problems and political considerations are minimized, but achievement of consensus can be effectively stymied when this is overdone. Team sizes should range from five to ten people.

To aid in team roster selection, we recommend that the team leader write down the name of the product or service to be improved or newly introduced. Then the team leader, and perhaps the sponsor, should do a rough block diagram — a high-level flow chart — of the complete process by which this product or service will be produced, indicating which departments or units are responsible for doing the work in each block.

Next, indicate which organization(s) are responsible for providing important elements in the work environment for the various

| PHASE I PLANNING |
| --- |
| **Step 1:** Organizing the Project |
| **Step 2:** Identifying Best Practitioners |
| **Step 3:** Preparing to Collect Data |

| PHASE I PLANNING |
| --- |
| Step 1: Organizing the Project |
| Step 2: Identifying Best Practitioners |
| Step 3: Preparing to Collect Data |

blocks. (For example, in the Blood Bank case, the engineering department was responsible for maintaining the blood products pneumatic tube transport system, and was therefore represented on the team.)

Finally, identify the group or groups who will be the major recipients of the product or service, and any other major stakeholders, whether internal or external.

A frequent problem with benchmarking projects is that the extent of the required changes is underestimated. More often than not there is a **ripple effect**: a change in one of your work processes will necessitate changes in the way things are done by people in some other service who receive your output, or provide your inputs, or contribute in some way to supporting your work environment. For example, in the Blood Bank case, one recommendation was that the engineers who supported the pneumatic tube system make some important changes in blood product carriers. Had they not been represented on the project team, their cooperation might have been harder to get.

The ripple effect is particularly important in the case of a new product or service, where it is not always possible, even with a good imagination, to foresee all the interactions that the new entity will have with the existing order of things. In this situation, it is wise to err on the side of inclusiveness.

A few rules of thumb in making up the team roster are:

- Always include members from the organizations with the most detailed knowledge of the most important subject matter.

- Always include members from the organizations likely to have the greatest role in carrying out the recommendations. (This could require adding a member after the project is under way, which is undesirable, but better than risking problems at the end of the project. For example, at the end of the Stroke Therapy Initiative case in Part II, the team lost time because they didn't know who should do some of the work they were recommending.)

- Try to include representatives from organizations that will be directly affected by the changes in work flow likely to be recommended by the team — e.g., the customers of the output of the changed work processes. For example, in the Blood Bank case, a nurse supervisor from a unit that uses a lot of blood products is on the team.

- If a subject is particularly sensitive politically, it is sometimes expedient to take this into consideration in selecting team members. These situations must be handled in an *ad hoc* way.

- A manageable size for a benchmarking team is usually six to eight members.

- In order to keep teams to a manageable size, consider using internal consultants and advisors with important information on specialized topics as **guest experts** at meetings where their topic is being discussed.

| PHASE I PLANNING |
| --- |
| Step 1: Organizing the Project |
| Step 2: Identifying Best Practitioners |
| Step 3: Preparing to Collect Data |

## BUILDING THE TEAM

Once the individual participants have been recruited, the best way to build them into a team is to put the group to work immediately on meaningful project activities. By focusing on what brought the group *together*, attention is automatically led away from what might keep them *apart*. A good sequence might be:

- Discuss and refine the goal of the project based on a better understanding of how it supports the overall objective.

- Develop team self-governance procedures — how to run the team meetings, attendance rules, etc.

- Learn tools and techniques that will be needed immediately in the project — e.g., brainstorming/ways to organize ideas, how to reach consensus, methods of data analysis, etc. (Optional or as-required for an institution practicing TQM/CQI.)

For more information and ideas about what to do to bring a team up to speed quickly, see the first appendix on Team Building.

PHASE I
PLANNING

Step 1:
Organizing
the Project

Step 2:
Identifying Best
Practitioners

Step 3:
Preparing to
Collect Data

## DEVELOPING A TEAM CHARTER

The benchmarking team should begin thinking about its charter, or contract with the sponsor, immediately. However, it should not prepare this document until it has achieved a detailed understanding of what the project is all about. This seldom happens at the first team meeting.

The team leader and sponsor can help focus the team's attention on the right topics by preparing a draft of the charter and giving it to the team for study and critique. For an example of a team charter, see the Blood Bank case, Figure 8.

The team charter should contain:

- Project scope and constraints. The **project scope** defines the subject matter the project is expected to address. This is not just a formality. All activities in an organization are linked to other activities and are embedded in the organization's working environment. It is sometimes hard to tell where the boundaries of the project's scope should be. The charter document helps to keep things on track. For example, in the Stroke Therapy Initiative case in Part II, the team's scope is to study *how to introduce* a new protocol. The team loses track of its scope and begins developing the protocol itself, duplicating the work of another project in the overall stroke initiative program. The charter is used to remind the group of what they have been asked to do.

  **Constraints** refer to limitations on what the sponsor can commit to on his or her side of the bargain. For example, a constraint might be that no recommendations are acceptable that call for a capital expenditure of more than $xx.

- Requirements for success. (See Step 3, p. 27 for a definition of these measures.)

- Resources. Roster of team members and their time commitment; authorized expenditures by the team, including travel; training and facilitator support; etc.

16

- Output. Definition of the project report contents: action recommendations, due date, and sometimes an implementation plan.
- Team schedule.

**Note:** Throughout Step 1 activity, and throughout the entire project, the sponsor has an ongoing responsibility to cultivate and maintain the support of management and the major stakeholders.

| PHASE I PLANNING |
| --- |
| Step 1: Organizing the Project |
| Step 2: Identifying Best Practitioners |
| Step 3: Preparing to Collect Data |

# STEP 2: IDENTIFYING THE BEST PRACTITIONERS

The formal and informal networks of professional specialists give healthcare an advantage over many industrial companies in Step 2. In organizations as diverse as the American Academy of Physician Executives and the American Association of Blood Banks, healthcare workers are linked by nationwide ties based on devotion to their various specialties.

These ties make the search for best practitioners and suitable benchmarking partners a great deal easier. They may be used in two distinct ways: the self-initiated approach and the group-initiated approach, as discussed below. The *substance* of what must be done remains the same, however, and will be discussed first.

## POSITIONING THE PROJECT

The overall project objective may be to improve performance in an already established service or to obtain help starting a new service. In either case, the team will need to be honest with itself about the organization's current performance level, its ambitions, and its ability to commit resources. Generally, institutions with high performance levels seem ambitious enough to go even higher or to try new things, and are willing to commit the resources necessary to do so. Unfortunately, the converse often seems to be true as well. *Know thyself* is a valuable injunction at this point. It will save a great deal of wasted motion.

PHASE I
PLANNING

Step 1:
Organizing
the Project

Step 2:
Identifying Best
Practitioners

Step 3:
Preparing to
Collect Data

We offer two rules of thumb, one for each of the extremes:

1. Modest goals. Best for organizations uncomfortable with major changes and having very limited resources for benchmarking. If you are seeking quick and/or inexpensive results, consider looking close to home initially. If you can learn from the person in the next-door office, or in another department of your organization, do so. This approach is commonly called *internal benchmarking*, and can be both productive and cost-effective when done carefully. It obviously is inappropriate for initiating new services.

2. Ambitious goals. Best for organizations that are seriously contemplating radical change in their approach and/or are already leaders in the area under scrutiny. Going further afield makes you more apt to encounter better practices, of course. "World-class" and "best-of-the-best" performances can be located only by literally searching worldwide. Major cost-reduction and reengineering programs are best supported by this style of benchmarking.

Most organizations fall between these extremes, and the decision on how far afield to go will depend partly on your relative standing. For example, if you know that your organization's performance is well below the national median in an area, there is (by definition) a more than 50-50 chance that an organization chosen completely at random can offer a degree of incremental help.

Your decision about how widely to cast your net will always be situational, however, driven by such considerations as the severity and urgency of the problems being studied, whether you are contemplating a new service or an improved one, availability of contacts, travel budgets, time constraints, etc.

## SEEKING BENCHMARKING PARTNER SOURCES

In the search for suitable **benchmarking partners**, a benchmarking team can make its own list of sources, or it can consider groups set up for this purpose. The two approaches are not equivalent, however, and need separate discussion.

18

**Note:** You are only ready to make tentative *contacts* at this point! See "Recruiting Benchmarking Partners" on page 32.

### The self-initiated approach.

This approach may be indicated when your organization has established a well-defined objective (e.g., develop new products and services) and wishes to benchmark a particular subject (e.g., liver transplant) related to that objective. Some pointers are:

- All benchmarking team members should contribute to a list of potential partners. Other stakeholders and opinion-makers should also be solicited for ideas.

- Use all available resources to find potential partners, including professional contacts, the literature, and material from conferences and conventions.

- Regardless of how widely the informal search for benchmarking partners extends, be sure to learn as much relevant information as possible about potential partners before you make formal contact. For example, the size of the other organization, how many beds it has if it is a hospital, types of care provided, etc., are all items of information that can usually be obtained from publicly available sources. If you decide that some characteristic of the organization is important to your study, look for it in these resources first.

- Generally, benchmarking *partnership* means that full reciprocity is offered and accepted. Thus, any information requested in a questionnaire must also be offered by your institution in exchange; an invitation for a site visit should be reciprocated, and so on. How much you are willing to share with your benchmarking partners can have an important bearing on whether you want to partner with them. (For a discussion of how to circumvent the problem of *secrecy* between organizations in competition with one another, see Chapter 10.)

- Decide how many benchmarking partners you wish to include in your project. This will have an impact on the type of questionnaire you prepare, the data tabulation, and

| PHASE I |
| PLANNING |
| Step 1: Organizing the Project |
| Step 2: Identifying Best Practitioners |
| Step 3: Preparing to Collect Data |

PHASE I
PLANNING

Step 1:
Organizing
the Project

Step 2:
Identifying Best
Practitioners

Step 3:
Preparing to
Collect Data

how you prepare the report in which you compare institutions. If you have a small number of partners, four, for example (a typical number), it is customary to provide each with a report identifying your organization and that of the partner receiving the report, with the other partners identified only by a code.

Another very effective way to identify possible partners is through contacts made at national conferences organized by various groups. Some notable examples include:

**The Institute for Healthcare Improvement** (IHI). In addition to its activities mentioned in the Introduction, the IHI also conducts an annual National Forum on Quality Improvement in Health Care, and teaches a variety of courses emphasizing quality improvement measures.

**The Healthcare Forum.** This publisher of the *Healthcare Forum Journal* conducts applied research in healthcare policy issues and sponsors educational seminars on a variety of topics of interest to both administrators and clinicians.

Some of your informal searches for benchmarking partner candidates may very likely take place *via* the Internet. In fact, occasionally, the entire project may be carried out this way. A discussion of how the Internet affects the benchmarking phases may be found in Chapter 9.

## The group-initiated approach.

This approach is indicated if your organization has an ongoing interest in an area where there is already an established interest group. By joining the group, an institution can determine its relative standing with respect to the other members of the group, and frequently obtain generally useful descriptions of best practices from leaders in the field. If resources are scarce and there is a sufficiently close overlap of interests, what this approach may lack in opportunity for in-depth probing it may make up in convenience; minimal use of your own people's time, and frequently low cost. Different kinds of group-initiated benchmarking efforts have different characteristics, however, and the selection should be made based on your own needs. Examples are described below.

**The American Academy of Pediatrics** (AAP). The AAP conducts a program designed to enable physicians in both individual and group practice to improve the quality of patient care. The Ambulatory Care Quality Improvement Program, or ACQIP, makes it possible for physicians to compare their practices with those of other physicians participating in the program.

Since 1991, the ACQIP has carried out over 25 studies in a range of topics related to the interests of Academy members. These studies (called "Exercises" by the AAP) involve participants who answer a set of questions, do chart reviews, and complete patient satisfaction surveys about how they conduct their own practice. The results are compiled and returned to the participants in such a manner that each participating practice can compare its answers with those of the population of respondents, up to 3,000 nationwide in the USA on the state, district, and national levels.

In addition to the reports, participants also receive clinical practice guidelines and/or practice parameters where applicable, and a collection of quality pointers, including literature reviews, "pearls of wisdom" from other respected practitioners, and listings of other sources of information concerning best practices.

Participation in the exercises earns the individual member appropriate CME credits in either the AAP or the American Academy of Family Physicians as well as Risk Management credits.

**The College of American Pathologists** (CAP). The CAP conducts the Q-Probes Program, which is a benchmarking program for pathology and laboratory medicine. Its objective is "to evaluate factors that affect laboratory performance and to benchmark quality indicators for all phases of the testing and reporting process."

Beginning in 1989, the Q-Probes Program has carried out approximately 80 studies through year-end 1996. The program has compiled a substantial database from a variety of institutions, including laboratories serving small and large hospitals and outpatient settings. In addition to the Q-Probes reports, which are avail-

| PHASE I PLANNING |
| --- |
| Step 1: Organizing the Project |
| Step 2: Identifying Best Practitioners |
| Step 3: Preparing to Collect Data |

PHASE I
PLANNING

Step 1:
Organizing
the Project

Step 2:
Identifying Best
Practitioners

Step 3:
Preparing to
Collect Data

able from the CAP, an impressive collection of publications has appeared in the referenced literature. (R. B. Schifman *et al.*, 1996)

**The International Benchmarking Clearinghouse.** This division of the American Productivity & Quality Center (APQC), a nonprofit education and research organization serving all sectors of the business world, has a membership of over 400 companies, many engaged in activities directly involved with healthcare. It carries out Consortium Benchmarking Studies on a variety of topics of general interest to the membership. It also will do studies on topics requested by one or a group of members.

**The Institute for Healthcare Improvement.** This institute carries out a number of topical studies each year, with 20 to 40 participating organizations. The purpose of these "collaboratives" is for the participants to learn from each other and from outstanding leaders in the field. There is strong emphasis on putting what is learned into practice. Recent studies have included: Improving Asthma Care in Children and Adults, and Reducing Adverse Drug Events and Medical Errors.

**Consulting firms.** Over time, most consulting firms will build up a substantial library of completed reports from their own self-initiated studies. Sometimes it is possible to locate and purchase exactly what you want by searching the catalogues of these collections. In that sense, a consultant's library is in the same category as other libraries to be searched at the outset of your project.

There are many consulting firms, some small, some very large, which are capable of organizing and conducting new inquiries on behalf of a group of clients interested in a particular topic. These "multi-client studies," as they are called, have certain advantages. For example, vending firms are responsible for finding suitable participants. Also, these studies are commonly structured to preserve the anonymity of all participants, and most organizations seem to be more willing to divulge confidential information under this condition. However, you may want to ask detailed follow-up questions, frequently on a face-to-face basis, but that compromises the agreement to preserve anonymity.

# STEP 3: PREPARING TO COLLECT DATA

The discussion in Step 3 focuses on projects whose goal is to improve the performance of an existing process. The ideas are also applicable to developing a new service, with some modifications.

## FLOW-CHARTING THE PROCESS

Remember the Golden Rule of TQM/CQI (p.5): *The way to improve an output is to improve the process that produces the output.*

Improving a work process starts with knowing what it is. Most work processes in most organizations are not described in detail. This is no longer as true in healthcare as it was a decade ago, thanks to the advent of critical pathways, practice parameters, and the like. While many of the clinical protocols in patient care are now well documented, a great many of the clinical work processes, as well as those in the supporting environment, remain undocumented.

The best way to document a work process is to gather the people who know the most about the process (ideally the benchmarking team, plus perhaps a few other specialists) and build a flow-chart of the process. If one already exists, time should be spent reviewing its accuracy and completeness. Next, the completed flow-chart should always be reviewed by the **process owner** (the person accountable for the process and its output(s)) and her or his work group. If they are not satisfied that it fairly represents what they do, their cooperation later in shifting over to an improved process will be compromised.

Study of a completed process flow-chart usually produces both surprise and enlightenment. Typically, when first seeing the flow diagram of a moderately complicated work process laid out in some detail, people respond with, "Good Lord, is that what we do? No wonder we have so many problems!"

This instant reaction may be all the analysis needed to start the improvement cycle. It is often appropriate to fix glaring errors of omission, duplication of effort, and lack of communication immediately. Why labor over no-brainers?

| PHASE I PLANNING |
| --- |
| Step 1: Organizing the Project |
| Step 2: Identifying Best Practitioners |
| Step 3: Preparing to Collect Data |

PHASE I
PLANNING

Step 1:
Organizing
the Project

Step 2:
Identifying Best
Practitioners

Step 3:
Preparing to
Collect Data

Usually, however, the problems are more complex and subtle, requiring the detailed study and searching that benchmarking was designed to do.

## IDENTIFYING MEASURES OF QUALITY

Measures of quality are the basis for benchmarking comparisons. (Recall that **quality** simply means that a process does what it should do, and the output is what it should be.) Until these measures have been defined and ranked in importance, there is no way to tell whether one organization's performance is better or worse than another's. How can you decide which organization has better quality performance if you have no way of defining what "better" really means?

Measures all have two parts — the **metric** and the **value**. The metric is the unit of measure; the value is the amount of that unit. For example, the metric for a person's height is centimeters; for Joan the value may be 165; for John, 180. Good measures usually have metrics that lend themselves easily to the use of numerical values. However, this is not always the case, and the best test of a measure is whether it helps you separate the desirable from the less desirable in an objective way. For example, in the Blood Bank case it was important to know whether a potential benchmarking partner had a pneumatic tube transport system (the metric), and the answer was either yes or no; a binary *value*.

Good measures of quality make it easy to express **standards**. For example, a standard for inclusion on a basketball team might be that each player's weight be between 80 and 100 kilograms. Thus, an aspiring player's weight (the metric) might be 120 kilograms (the value), clearly showing that he does not meet the standard. (Note that using weight as one of the metrics for a measure of basketball-playing quality is a matter of choice. The coach's objective is to have a basketball team that is better than the competition, and he has *decided* that one of his measures of quality is "weight within a certain range." The point is that his choice of a metric and an associated value for it gives the coach an unambiguous standard for his chosen measure of quality.)

There are three kinds of measures of quality, and they are all important in a benchmarking project:

PHASE I
PLANNING

Step 1:
Organizing
the Project

Step 2:
Identifying Best
Practitioners

Step 3:
Preparing to
Collect Data

1. Measures of adherence to standard process. These measures allow monitoring of whether a prescribed set of steps for doing things exists and, if so, whether this prescribed way is being followed. Until recently, this was the most important measure of quality emphasized in accreditation surveys of healthcare organizations. Now there is a move to increase the emphasis on the other two kinds of measures.

2. Measures of output quality. These are measures that determine whether the required product was produced. For example, the crucial measure of output quality from the order-filling process in a pharmacy confirms that a prescription contains the correct dosage of the correct medication for the correct patient. More broadly, a crucial measure of output quality for a treatment protocol is *clinical outcome.*

3. Measures of in-process quality. As the name implies, these are measures that allow monitoring of the output during production to confirm that everything is on track to the required end-point. For example, in the pharmacy case above, one in-process measure is whether the correct patient number has been matched to the correct order number. As another example, one measure of in-process quality for a blood draw is whether the sample was drawn at the right time.

As with the flow-chart, the process owner and the work group responsible for carrying out the process should be asked to review the measures of quality for accuracy, usefulness, relevance, and, above all, fairness in monitoring the process as it is currently performed.

Once the flow-chart has been agreed to, the benchmarking team can identify and rank the measures of output quality that it wishes to emphasize in its search for better performance. This

**PHASE I
PLANNING**

**Step 1:
Organizing
the Project**

**Step 2:
Identifying Best
Practitioners**

**Step 3:
Preparing to
Collect Data**

requires a certain amount of fearlessness, because it will be necessary to acknowledge performance shortfalls that some individuals or organizations may wish to forget. But it has to be done.

Next, the team will need to identify the in-process quality measures that can be tied directly to output quality measures. This is not easy, partly because it is usually unfamiliar territory, but more importantly because the actual cause-and-effect relationships are often unknown. The problem of not being able to identify in-process quality measures is a fundamental issue for all organizations where there is a substantial time lag between what one does (the cause) and the outcome (the effect). Health care and education at all levels are particularly affected by this problem.

Industries where products are made under conditions where cause-and-effect relationships are not well understood are said to produce "products by process," and the process is often simply a recipe that has always worked. It is nevertheless still possible to have in-process measures that check to see whether the recipe is being followed faithfully. In the bakery industry, for example, getting a flaky piecrust requires using cold water in the mix. Perhaps no one really understands the physical chemistry of why this is so, but the water temperature can still be measured.

Finding out how tenuous our understanding is of some of the supposed cause-and-effect relationships is often the starting point for some of the most productive lines of inquiry in a benchmarking project. For example, if an organization does not know the relationship between the length of in-service training in phlebotomy and competent performance as a phlebotomist, cross-training of other personnel can go badly astray. Benchmarking comparisons with partner organizations can be a fruitful line of inquiry in such a case.

Finally, the team needs to assess candidly just how strict is the **adherence to the standard** — the process flow-chart. Here again, fearlessness will probably be called for. Often, the people who do

26

the actual work use various shortcuts and they see little point in mentioning this to other people, whom they may very well regard as outsiders and perhaps even meddlers.

## IDENTIFYING REQUIREMENTS FOR SUCCESS FOR THE PROJECT

Early in the project, frequently at the first team meeting, two related questions are almost inevitably asked:

"What are we *really* here for?"

"How will we know if our project has accomplished that?"

This is your opportunity to begin tying the overall objective of the benchmarking project — which should be stated in rather general terms at this point — to the **requirements for success** of the project. Requirements for success must be sharply worded statements about things that can be measured with some precision. Usually the best way to do this is to start by identifying a short list of quantitative facts you must learn in order to meet your objective.

For example, in the Blood Bank case, the overall objective is to improve the operation of the blood bank, and one of the requirements for success is to provide data on the range of blood product delivery times achievable by the best practitioners.

Usually factual information about five to ten crucial measures of quality are required in order to characterize how well the work processes and outputs of your operation stack up against those of the best organizations available to you for comparison. Once these have been listed, the requirements for success for the project fall into three main categories:

1. Getting the required information about the crucial measures of quality, usually in numerical form.

2. Finding out how superior results were achieved for the chosen measures of quality.

3. Successfully adopting or adapting the superior approach for use in your own operation.

PHASE I
PLANNING

Step 1:
Organizing
the Project

Step 2:
Identifying Best
Practitioners

Step 3:
Preparing to
Collect Data

| PHASE I PLANNING |
| :---: |
| **Step 1:** Organizing the Project |
| **Step 2:** Identifying Best Practitioners |
| **Step 3:** Preparing to Collect Data |

In the early days of benchmarking, some argued that the only thing a benchmarking project should do is to find how much better the competition is; the job of finding out *how the results were achieved* should be left as a challenge to the people accountable for these results in their own organization. However, it was soon discovered that neither the benchmarkers, management, or the accountable workers were satisfied with this approach. Everyone wanted to know immediately what should be done about the challenge. It became apparent that the way to do this was to deal with all aspects of the situation at once, and to involve the people who would have to develop a workable response to the challenge intimately in the benchmarking process.

## USING INFORMATION SOURCES

Information needed for a benchmarking project can often be found by searching through the library. (The term *library* includes all organized information sources, including those accessed *via* the Internet.) The information will be useful in two ways in the search for benchmarking partners: it helps identify them, and it facilitates the first contact when you decide to approach them. Knowing something about the person on the other end of the phone line always makes initial contact easier.

Use the library intelligently. If there are librarians (including web browsers and search engines, those somewhat inadequate Internet surrogates for librarians), don't hesitate to get help.

Be imaginative. A reasonably uninhibited search can trigger new thoughts that may enrich your view of your problem. Don't go too far out, though. Project teams tend to stray beyond their intended scope anyhow, and far-fetched connections only raise the noise level of a project meeting.

Every field has its special sources. In the industrial world, SEC filings, 10K reports, and the like are useful sources. In clinical medicine, the compilations of practice parameters published by the Practice Parameter Partnership are a rich source of information and ideas. The same may be said for the Clinical Practice Guideline series published by the U.S. Department of Health and Human Services' Agency for Health Care Policy and Research. Both of these sources follow high standards of scholarship and consensus development.

A more controversial type of source is the outcomes compilations produced by various state agencies. The New York State Cardiac Surgery Reporting System and the reports of the Pennsylvania Health Care Cost Containment Council are examples. However problematic they may be at present, with questions about the burdensome cost of reporting, validity of the risk-adjustment methodology, etc., outcomes measures and compilations of indicator measurements will inevitably become more common. These databases are thought by some knowledgeable observers to show considerable promise as future sources of useful benchmarking information (Brennan and Berwick 1996, 203).

In this connection, the work of the Joint Commission on Accreditation of Healthcare Organizations (JCAHO) in the development and extension of its *Indicator Measurement System*, or IMSystem, deserves special mention. In 1987 the JCAHO embarked on its "Agenda for Change," an ambitious, multifaceted program with an objective of shifting the emphasis of its activities from Quality Assurance to Quality Improvement. One major element of this program was the IMSystem, which has been in development since 1989 and is being implemented in a growing number of hospitals.

The IMSystem includes 31 clinical indicators apportioned by the following areas: anesthesia-related (2), obstetrics/gyn (5), cardiovascular (5), oncology (5), trauma (6), medicinal usage (5), and infection control (3). All of these indicators were developed with major participation of practicing clinicians. Some are focused on *in-process performance measures* (time elapsed from arrival in the Emergency Department to commencement of thrombolytic treatment in the case of acute heart attack) and others on *outcomes measures* (complications within two postoperative days following anesthesia).

| PHASE I PLANNING |
| --- |
| Step 1: Organizing the Project |
| Step 2: Identifying Best Practitioners |
| Step 3: Preparing to Collect Data |

PHASE I
PLANNING

Step 1:
Organizing
the Project

Step 2:
Identifying Best
Practitioners

Step 3:
Preparing to
Collect Data

Participants in the IMSystem submit data to a central location where it is compiled and analyzed statistically. Individual hospitals receive quarterly reports showing their own results on tables, bar graphs, and control charts against the aggregated results for all other participants in the system. The data are risk-adjusted for the individual patient episode and also adjusted for hospital characteristics in the population of participating hospitals. Your hospital's actual performance for the period is thus compared on an adjusted basis with your predicted performance for each of the reported indicators.

When looked at from a benchmarking perspective, it is clear that the IMSystem addresses one of the objectives of the benchmarking process: it enables an organization to find out how it stacks up against the aggregate population of its peers. In the present stage of development of the IMSystem, it is not yet possible to directly compare with the performance of the best performers, or to learn how they achieved their superior results. However, these are early days in what must be recognized as a monumental undertaking.

In early 1996, the Joint Commission announced a plan to create a National Library of Healthcare Indicators (NLHI). The intention is that the NLHI will include indicators that have been developed through the Agency for Health Care Policy and Research, the National Committee for Quality Assurance, Kaiser Permanente, and many others. This emphasis on a consensual approach may lead to long-term success in providing the responsible outcomes reporting system demanded by the public, while also being useful for sharing best practices within the healthcare community itself. We believe it to be consistent with the spirit of the concepts of *enforced self-regulation and responsive regulation* (Ayres and Braithwaite, 1992, 4).

## DEVELOPING QUESTIONNAIRES

A benchmarking team should get as much information as possible using the sources and methods described above. At some point, however, it will be necessary to ask specific questions of the benchmarking partners, customarily using questionnaires. When developing such questionnaires, it is wise to remember that people are "questionnaired" to death these days, and do not take kindly to poorly designed examples of the *genre*. Keep it as short, to-the-point, and as user-friendly as possible. A detailed discussion of how to develop a questionnaire is found in Appendix 2.

There are four kinds of information you need to find out in a benchmarking project:

| PHASE I PLANNING |
| --- |
| Step 1: Organizing the Project |
| Step 2: Identifying Best Practitioners |
| Step 3: Preparing to Collect Data |

1. **Partnership potential information.** This information establishes that the other organization would be a suitable benchmarking partner. The questions you will need to ask are called "**screener**" questions, and they will go into a **screener questionnaire**. The questions are ones that you probably cannot answer with library-type searches and include queries about such things as the existence of a database of performance, recent trends in performance, willingness to cooperate, etc.

The main project questionnaire seeks the following detailed information:

2. **Performance information.** This information provides the basis for comparing your institution's performance with the best practitioners. The questions are ones the benchmarking team was chartered to answer, and are derived directly from the first category — measures of quality — of the team's requirements for success, with perhaps some elaboration of the context of the question. If benchmarking partners have been chosen well, they will understand the questions and be willing and able to supply answers.

3. **Work process information.** This information reveals how the other organization has achieved its superior performance. These questions are also ones that the benchmarking team was chartered to answer, and are derived directly from the second category of the team's requirements for success. They will start you on the path to learning how your partners achieve their enviable results.

31

PHASE I
PLANNING

Step 1:
Organizing
the Project

Step 2:
Identifying Best
Practitioners

Step 3:
Preparing to
Collect Data

4. **Work environment information.** This information, also derived directly from the second category of the team's requirements for success, helps in understanding the support structures and culture of the other organization. The questions concern details of factors in the other organization's environment that could have a major impact on how effective their work processes are. For example, in the blood bank case, the team needs to know key details about the organizational responsibility for maintenance of the blood products pneumatic tube transport system that is used by its partners.

When developing a questionnaire, all members of the team should be encouraged to participate by submitting possible questions. However, questionnaires can be a nightmare, and if possible, you should always take advantage of people who have some experience. For example, the Marketing Department may be able to help in questionnaire construction. Further discussion of how to develop a questionnaire may be found in Appendix 2.

## RECRUITING BENCHMARKING PARTNERS

As many members of the benchmarking team as feasible should participate in partner recruitment. Those who may have made some initial informal contacts in Step 2 should follow up by doing the recruiting.

All partner recruiting, which is ordinarily done by telephone, should be done using the screener questionnaire. Decision-critical items in the candidate profile, which are already known from library-type inquiries, should be *validated* at this time — It will both ensure accuracy and serve as a subtle form of flattery to the potential partners when you demonstrate considerable knowledge of their institutions.

If the original informal contact was with a personal acquaintance, or if there has been no actual contact previous to the recruiting call, it is likely that the first call will not put you in touch with the right person. Quickly explain what your call is about, and ask who would be the right person in the candidate organization for you to talk with. It can take as many as three calls to get to the right person, but the effort is worthwhile.

PHASE I
PLANNING

Step 1:
Organizing
the Project

Step 2:
Identifying Best
Practitioners

Step 3:
Preparing to
Collect Data

Once you have reached the right person — one who is in the function you are concerned about and is in a position to commit to participation — explain what you are trying to do, and what would be involved. Use the screener questionnaire to establish the desirability of the candidate as a benchmarking partner, and use your best selling skills to make them want to join your effort.

Usually a potential partner will not be very interested in how *you* do the work in question — after all, they get better results than you do! However, if you explain that they will have access to the performance of other, suitably identity-disguised participants, experience has shown that a high level of interest can be expected. Also, stress that there may be an opportunity for reciprocity or barter: they may well be interested in how your organization performs some other task, and this can be a satisfactory basis for partnership. For example, in the Blood Bank case study, one of the benchmarking partners was interested in learning about some aspects of starting an organ transplant program. (Be careful you don't promise a barter that you can't complete, however!)

In recruiting calls, here are a few things to keep in mind:

- Explain upfront who you are and what your intentions are. This is the benchmarker's code of ethics in a nutshell.

- Use your screener questionnaire in a conversational way.

- Promise feedback in the form of a useful report.

- Promise an opportunity for a return visit in case a site visit becomes appropriate. (First make sure you can deliver.)

- Do not disguise the amount of work involved. If the questionnaire is long, explain that it will take a nontrivial amount of time to complete it, but that it is intentionally constructed so that no one person will have the burden of answering the whole questionnaire.

- Find out if there will be a fee for services.

PHASE I
PLANNING

Step 1:
Organizing
the Project

Step 2:
Identifying Best
Practitioners

Step 3:
Preparing to
Collect Data

After all the screening calls have been completed, the results should be tabulated and circulated to the team as homework. At the next team meeting, a short list of key discriminants for the most desirable partners should be developed and the candidates scored. Such things as performance level, willingness to participate, proximity, etc., might be on the list of discriminants. If the initial search for potential partners was well done, at least 40% of the list will be highly desirable, based on these discriminants. For an example of the use of this approach, see Table 1 in the Blood Bank case.

The selected partners should be notified and confirmed immediately, and told that the next step will be for them to receive and fill out the questionnaire.

## ANSWERING YOUR OWN QUESTIONNAIRE

Many people are tempted to skip this step. We feel it is essential, however, for a number of reasons:

- It establishes the official baseline for your own performance in metrics that are understood and accepted by the people who do the work.

- It gives the people who are responsible for the processes and outputs under study another opportunity to participate. Their review of the flow-chart and the measures of quality has already made them familiar with the project's intentions. Now they will have the chance to make a direct contribution to the establishment of a baseline for comparison with the benchmarking partners.

- You have agreed to trade results with your benchmarking partners.

- It is the best way to do a final try-out or "pilot" of the questionnaire under realistic conditions before taking it on the road. To avoid loss of time, it can be done simultaneously with benchmarking partner recruiting.

34

*When you are able to answer your own questionnaire, particularly when you can provide a process flow diagram and numerical data for the measures of quality, you will have realized much of the benefit of a benchmarking project.*

| PHASE I PLANNING |
| --- |
| Step 1: Organizing the Project |
| Step 2: Identifying Best Practitioners |
| Step 3: Preparing to Collect Data |

You have now completed Phase I and are ready to begin your data collection fieldwork.

## Checklist for a Successful Phase I

- Clear purpose stated.
- Important subject chosen.
- Project scope clearly defined.
- All key stakeholders identified.
- Strong management support obtained.
- Strong, motivated team leader recruited.
- Strong group of people with the right skills and affiliations recruited.
- Cohesive, motivated team built.
- Tightly focused set of measures of project success developed.
- Measures of quality tied tightly to the project's requirements for success chosen.
- Clear, stable team charter established.
- Benchmarking partner candidate list prepared and rated.
- Benchmarking partners recruited.
- Questionnaire based on the measures of quality and the other measures of success developed.
- Questionnaire piloted in-house by the people who do the work.

*Make sure that everything you have done so far is self-consistent.*

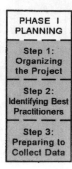

## Possible Phase I Pitfalls

### Step 1: Organizing the Project

- No clear purpose
- Unimportant subject, wrong subject, diffuse subject(s)
- "Ripple-effect" changes not identified
- Poor team balance
- Poorly chosen metrics, too many/too few metrics
- Poorly prepared team charter
- Lukewarm management support

### Step 2: Identifying the Best Practitioners

- In-house learning opportunities ignored
- Leading institutions not considered
- Personal contacts not used

### Step 3: Preparing to Collect Data

- Inadequate use of publicly available information
- Poorly thought-out questions
- Questionnaire not piloted in-house
- Benchmarking partners not fully informed of what partnership entails

# Chapter 2

---

# Phase II: Data Collection and Analysis

---

*Phase II begins with detailed information-gathering
and concludes with the emergence of a possible set of
recommended actions and improvement goals based
on the benchmarking team's findings.*

Along the way you will answer a number of key questions:

> Why is it better to have our benchmarking partners
> answer our questionnaire by mail?
>
> What must we think about if we wish to administer our
> questionnaire by phone?
>
> What do we do first when we get the questionnaires
> back?
>
> Why can questionnaire administration by E-mail be
> advantageous?
>
> How do we prepare for an efficient team discussion based
> on the findings?
>
> What should the team accomplish in the meeting to
> discuss the findings?

What is the **gap profile**, and why is it important to treat this information as confidential at this stage?

What should we be asking ourselves about the **best practices** we identify in our findings?

How do we start developing **improvement goals**?

How do we start turning our **findings** into **recommended actions**?

What is a **gap projection** and how do we make one?

What must we watch out for if we wish to adopt *all* of the good ideas we have gathered?

How do we determine if site visits are needed?

How do we ensure a successful site visit?

What if we are forced to combine administration of the questionnaire with a site visit?

At the conclusion of Phase II, the team will be ready to approach management to obtain support for its recommended actions.

| PHASE II DATA COLLECTION/ ANALYSIS |
| --- |
| Step 4: Administering Questionnaire |
| Step 5: Analyzing the Data |
| Step 6: Identifying Best Practices |
| Step 7: Doing Site Visits |

# STEP 4: ADMINISTERING THE QUESTIONNAIRE

There are two basic ways to administer the questionnaire — written and verbal. They share the same purpose, however: to obtain needed information about the benchmarking partners' performance and to determine how that performance was achieved. Benchmarking projects can vary considerably in scope and complexity, which should be taken into consideration when deciding which approach to follow.

## FULL-SCALE WRITTEN QUESTIONNAIRES (50–100+ITEMS)

Ordinarily, the best way to administer a written questionnaire is to have the partner organization fill it out without your presence. There are a number of reasons why this is so:

- It is cheaper. If you don't have to be there, no travel money needs to be spent at this stage.

- If your questionnaire is designed so that it requires your presence to get answers, it probably isn't thought out well enough and not ready for use.

- Your respondent will probably have to do some digging to retrieve some of the quantitative information, and your presence is a hindrance.

- If your questionnaire is well designed, your respondent will be able to distribute different sections to different people to answer. If you are present, this can cause scheduling problems.

PHASE II
DATA
COLLECTION/
ANALYSIS

Step 4:
Administering
Questionnaire

Step 5:
Analyzing the
Data

Step 6:
Identifying
Best Practices

Step 7: Doing
Site Visits

Alert your partner when you have sent out the questionnaire. Follow up with a phone call to encourage its immediate attention. When the document is sent electronically, be aware that formatting can get mangled by the Internet, and there is nothing more irritating than chaotic formatting in a questionnaire. You have gone to considerable pains to make the formatting user-friendly, and incompatible data-handling protocols can destroy this good work instantly.

Ask the recipient if the questions are clear and easily understood. Draw attention to the fact that the document is structured so that several people can work on different sections simultaneously. Emphasize that your team is standing by to answer any questions. If suitable, exchange names, phone numbers, e-mail addresses, etc., at this point, to encourage immediate attention to the response.

Make an agreement with your partners about a date when you can expect their responses. If this date arrives with no feedback, don't hesitate to follow up.

When the completed questionnaire is returned, look it over *immediately* to see whether any of the responses require clarification. The likelihood that obscure answers can be clarified is highest when the subject is still fresh in the mind of the respondent. Also, it demonstrates to your partners the importance you attach to the project.

## Short-Form Questionnaire (Less Than 40 Items)

If your questionnaire is short and narrowly focused on a specific topic, as in a "mini-benchmarking" project, you may wish to get the responses by telephone.

This approach may be desirable if there is great time urgency for completion of your benchmarking project. It has the advantage that partner response delays, due to more urgent priorities, procrastination, etc., are minimized. Also, clarification of obscure answers can take place on the spot, again reducing response turnaround time. Even here, however, it is helpful if your respondent has a chance to see the questionnaire, study it, and perhaps assemble some data *prior* to your interview call.

One disadvantage of the telephone interview is that there is a normal human tendency to stray from the appointed script to explore interesting details and side issues of mutual concern. When this happens, available time (and attention span!) may be used up before the whole questionnaire is covered.

Other disadvantages are that the responses may be less well thought through, the person asking the questions may bias the answers by unconscious verbal cues, and the responses may not be accurately recorded. Obviously, you will forego the advantage of having your respondents do the data entry as well. These problems are all sufficiently important to the quality of the study that you will want to think about them carefully before choosing to use the telephone conference approach to filling out your questionnaire.

Occasionally, and despite your best efforts, it may become necessary to combine completion of the questionnaire with a site visit. This is most likely to happen when there has been significant schedule slippage in Phase I. What to do in situations of this sort will be discussed in Step 7, Doing the Site Visit.

# STEP 5: ANALYZING THE DATA

## Compiling the Responses

The best way to compile responses to the questionnaire is to group all the answers to the same question, preferably in tabular

---

PHASE II
DATA
COLLECTION/
ANALYSIS

Step 4:
Administering
Questionnaire

Step 5:
Analyzing the
Data

Step 6:
Identifying
Best Practices

Step 7: Doing
Site Visits

---

form, with all the answers from respondent A in column A. A typical format for the compilation may be found in Table 2 of the Blood Bank case. The amount of time and effort required to complete this task is strictly dependent upon the nature of the questionnaire. Questionnaires that contain a lot of open-ended questions inviting essay-type responses will obviously require significantly more time than those with multiple or forced choices. In a typical situation with four benchmarking partners and an 80-item questionnaire with no more than 10 open-ended questions, it should take one person two to four hours to complete the tabulation by hand.

If the questionnaire was sent electronically and the responses were also made this way, compilation time can be shortened significantly, especially for the essay-type responses. With either approach, the task of compilation may be delegated to a nonteam member clerical person who can be trusted to be discreet (more about this later in the discussion of the gap-profile).

| PHASE II |
| DATA |
| COLLECTION/ |
| ANALYSIS |
| Step 4: |
| Administering |
| Questionnaire |
| Step 5: |
| Analyzing the |
| Data |
| Step 6: |
| Identifying |
| Best Practices |
| Step 7: Doing |
| Site Visits |

## IDENTIFYING THE BENCHMARKS AND GAP PROFILE

The next job is to analyze the tabulated responses for team study and discussion. This work should always be done by a team member, because detailed knowledge of the issues is necessary. The following activities are involved:

a. Go over the work to catch any ambiguities or qualifying notations to a multiple or forced-choice response. For example, in the answer to a multiple-choice question about how tissue samples are transported from the operating room to the pathology lab, the respondent may have checked "other," but supplied no further information. This type of reply will require follow-up by phone or e-mail for clarification.

b. All of the open-ended questions need study, particularly if the responses were tabulated by hand by a nonteam member. Be sure that the answer was transcribed without distortion. Identify, and note any common themes or similarities among the various answers to the same questions, and again look for answers with dubious meanings that may indicate additional follow-up.

c. This is also the place to do a reality check on whether the respondent's answers conform to the original profile you had envisioned, or even if they are really a suitable benchmarking partner. The screener is intended to ensure that this is not a problem, but examination of the full set of responses occasionally yields surprises. For example, during the screening call, the candidate benchmarking partner may have indicated that a computerized system for pharmacy order control was used, but the full questionnaire response reveals that the system is home-made, with lots of unmaintained code, and that several replacement approaches are being actively examined. This may change your views about how you wish to interact with this organization later.

d. For each key metric (number of patients tested per hour, cost of a procedure, percent of specimens labeled incorrectly, etc.) determine who is the best (the **benchmark**) among the respondents, and flag it for the team's attention. Usually you will find that no one respondent is the benchmark for all metrics.

e. If the team is benchmarking a process or service that your organization is currently practicing, determine, for each key metric, the **gap** between the benchmark performance and your own. If the key metrics have been carefully chosen and defined, this should be a number. For example, in the Blood Bank case study, average turnaround time for delivery of an order for a blood product was 45 minutes for the hospital doing the benchmarking project, while the benchmark was 26 minutes, resulting in a 19-minute gap. The whole set of performance gaps for the key metrics is called the **gap profile**. It is a summary picture of your organization's performance relative to benchmark performance, and tells at a glance where your

PHASE II
DATA
COLLECTION/
ANALYSIS

Step 4:
Administering
Questionnaire

Step 5:
Analyzing the
Data

Step 6:
Identifying
Best Practices

Step 7: Doing
Site Visits

organization stands with respect to the best available practices among your benchmarking partners.

If the subject of the benchmarking study is some new service your organization is considering, the set of benchmarks provides realistic performance goals for the individual metrics in that area. This information can greatly aid development planning of the new service.

**A word of caution:** Be very careful that all efforts to clarify ambiguous findings are directed to issues within the scope of the team charter. There is often a temptation to the compiler/analyst at this point to follow interesting leads suggested by the findings, but that go beyond the scope of the original intent. Don't succumb to this temptation. Your study was not designed to follow up extraneous leads, however interesting they may be. If they are followed, your time will be wasted, and of equal importance, the study's credibility will be compromised.

## REVIEWING THE FINDINGS

When these tasks are completed, the tabulated and annotated results, along with copies of the raw data, should be circulated to all team members for study.

After they have carefully studied the data compilation and analysis, team members are ready to meet to review and discuss what they have learned from the data-gathering questionnaire. The meeting agenda should cover the data, the analysis, the benchmarks, and, for services your organization provides now, the performance gap profile. Collectively, this package is called the **findings**, and it will become the factual basis for all subsequent actions. It is therefore vitally important to be sure that everyone on the team agrees with the findings — believes the data, understands the analysis, concurs in the benchmarks, and, for services your organization provides now, concurs in the performance gap profile. This is an ambitious goal for the meeting, and you may want to bring in a trained facilitator for the occasion.

The gap profile is often a mixed bag, with some good news and some bad, but it is a very sensitive collection of information,

| PHASE II DATA COLLECTION/ ANALYSIS |
| --- |
| Step 4: Administering Questionnaire |
| Step 5: Analyzing the Data |
| Step 6: Identifying Best Practices |
| Step 7: Doing Site Visits |

and must be treated accordingly. At this stage in the benchmarking project, it is good policy to treat the gap profile as confidential data, to be discussed only within the team. Taken out of context, without an understanding of the overall objective that the benchmarking project serves, and without any positive recommendations for action to offset the negative findings, news of the gap profile can become very corrosive grist for the rumor mill. There is a world of difference between "Have you heard that our returns to surgery are among the worst in the state?" and "I understand that there is a task force looking at ways to fix some problems we have with repeats on biopsies."

Great discretion is advised.

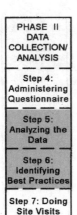

# STEP 6: IDENTIFYING BEST PRACTICES

In Step 5, team members studied, understood, and concurred on the **findings**. In Step 6, the team uses these findings to begin developing its recommendations. This step has three goals:

- To understand in detail how best practices work.
- To identify the greatest opportunities for improvement.
- To begin preparing conclusions and recommendations for action.

These goals are closely interwoven and should be reached through the best collective thinking of the team, which requires group interaction. The first two goals should be discussed together at a single team meeting. This makes for another ambitious agenda, but, as was the case in Step 5, thorough preparation for the meeting, and perhaps the use of a facilitator, can help to ensure success.

## UNDERSTANDING BEST PRACTICES

For each key metric, the benchmarking team needs to understand, in as much depth as possible, the practices that enabled the benchmark organization to achieve its superior results. Brief descriptions of these **best practices**, as determined from the questionnaire and any clarifying follow-up contacts, should be prepared and circulated to the entire team for individual study.

Divide this work up so that the descriptions are prepared in parallel by the most appropriate team members. This will make the effort less burdensome and save considerable time.

For each key metric (e.g., turnaround time for some category of biopsy or postoperative infection rate for a surgical procedure), the enabling best practice description should address:

- Important work process details.

- Essential details about the work environment. (For example, is it exceptionally supportive?)

- Considerations that might change interpretation of the comparison. (For example, does the benchmark organization refer exceptionally difficult cases elsewhere?)

- A draft of a **proposed set of actions** for your organization to carry out to achieve benchmark performance. This can be a good test of team understanding of a best practice, and it will be a useful starting point for preparing the team's conclusions and recommendations.

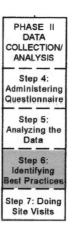

If an explanation of how a benchmarking partner *developed* a superior work process is available, it should also be included in the best practice description.

## IDENTIFYING OPPORTUNITIES

By now, team members should know from the circulated best practices descriptions what constitutes superior performance, how it was achieved (with perhaps some important details still missing), and how their own institution's performance compares, metric by metric. The stage is now set for a meeting-discussion based on fact about where the greatest opportunities lie, and what should be recommended to management. Because everyone in the group will want to give full attention to the substance (as opposed to the process) of this session, again it may be a good idea to bring in a dedicated facilitator for the occasion.

The central issue is how ambitious your recommendations should be for setting improvement goals for your institution. For example, is it possible for you or any other organization to be best in *all* the key metrics?

Do not leap to the conclusion that you can simply adopt the whole collection of approaches that enabled the other organizations individually to demonstrate benchmark performance for individual metrics. There may be incompatible circumstances that forbid going after everything. For example, one organization may achieve superior results for a given metric in a campus setting, while another organization shows superiority for a different metric in an urban high-rise environment. You would have to decide whether or not you can simultaneously adopt or adapt the different work processes that led to good results in these two quite different physical environments. If it is concluded that the differences are too great and you cannot follow two paths at once, a choice of which is more important must be made, or you must make tradeoffs which may give you better overall performance, yet still not be up to the individual benchmarks.

Occasionally, the team will find that there is a possibility of becoming the "best of the best" in your comparison universe. As a practical matter, however, the cost of such a move, both in financial terms and in terms of the organizational upheaval required, must be weighed against the benefits.

| PHASE II |
| DATA |
| COLLECTION/ |
| ANALYSIS |
| Step 4: Administering Questionnaire |
| Step 5: Analyzing the Data |
| Step 6: Identifying Best Practices |
| Step 7: Doing Site Visits |

## MAKING GAP PROJECTION

The discussion on improvement opportunities should address not only the current size of the gaps between your organization's performance and that of the benchmarks, but also what is likely to happen in the future. How fast will these gaps grow? Are the benchmark organizations resting on their laurels, or are they working on further improvements? If they continue to seek improvement, it is worthwhile to project the future course of their performance.

Rather than use valuable group meeting time to make these

projections, get the sense of the team's thinking and then delegate the making of the projections to the team members who prepared the best practice descriptions for each key metric. Some rules of thumb for this task are:

- Use simple assumptions and include them with the projections.
- Offer three versions of each projection — e.g., 5%, 10%, and 15% improvement in some metric over some time period.
- Note any evidence that the leaders are actively looking for ways to increase their lead.
- Emphasize what will happen to the gap if your organization does nothing.

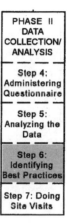

PHASE II
DATA
COLLECTION/
ANALYSIS

Step 4:
Administering
Questionnaire

Step 5:
Analyzing the
Data

Step 6:
Identifying
Best Practices

Step 7: Doing
Site Visits

If it becomes apparent during the discussion that the group is uncomfortable about its depth of understanding of one or more of the best practices, a site visit may be warranted. The main reason for a site visit is to find out things about how the organization to be visited gets its superior results, which are not adequately revealed in their answers to the questionnaire and in follow-up contacts. Site visits are not always needed, but if you have exhausted all other available means of getting required information, and there is no way to obtain the information you need short of seeing it for yourself, you have a good case for a site visit.

## PREPARING DRAFT RECOMMENDATIONS

You have now reached a critical point in the project. While the team is not yet ready to make a firm set of recommendations, its work to date needs to be boiled down into some summary conclusions. Here are two main reasons:

- The team needs to test how close to consensus its members are — the group needs to strike a *trial balance* on a proposed set of actions, to borrow a term from the accountants.
- The team needs a vehicle for communicating its views to the sponsor, the other stakeholders, and executive management.

- The group needs to float a *trial balloon*, to borrow a term from the politicians.

Team members who prepared the best practice descriptions for team discussion should summarize their work to date. Each topic should be covered briefly, with only enough detail to make a case for the proposed set of actions. These proposed actions should be essentially the same ones contained in the best practice description, modified by the team discussion. This activity can also be done in parallel to save time, with the individual drafts distributed to all team members for review.

At this point, the conclusions and recommendations should still be *tentative*. For example, if site visits are necessary, there may well be changes in your position as a result. Also, dialogue with the sponsor and others (see Phase IV) is likely to produce additional changes. Summarizing, Step 6 has accomplished three things:

- Best practices were understood.
- The greatest opportunities for improvement were considered.
- Assignments to prepare gap projections, summarize work to date, and draft preliminary recommendations were made.

Also, the need for a benchmarking partner site visit will have been considered.

## STEP 7: DOING SITE VISITS

The customary way to plan a site visit is for the prime contact on the benchmarking team to explore the possibility with the partner organization off-line and report back to the team. Be sure the partner understands the purpose of the visit. A major contributor to site visit success is clear agreement on the agenda by both the benchmarking team members and the people who will host the visit.

### PICKING A SITE VISIT SCENARIO

*Typical case.* The purpose of the visit is to extend and deepen your understanding of how your benchmarking partner has achieved

Sidebar:

PHASE II DATA COLLECTION/ ANALYSIS

Step 4: Administering Questionnaire

Step 5: Analyzing the Data

Step 6: Identifying Best Practices

Step 7: Doing Site Visits

superior results in particular areas. It builds on the knowledge obtained from study of the responses to your questionnaire and answers to questions for clarification raised in subsequent contacts by phone and/or e-mail. Thus, the visit should have an agenda that is tightly focused on a relatively few topics that you intend to explore to considerable depth. When this is clearly understood and agreed upon by both parties, the site visit should produce the desired outcome.

Because a visit to a given site will cover only particular topics, be sure that the individuals who make the visit are the right ones. For example, if the subject is specific to the pathology lab's work processes, do not send a specialist in computer software unless there is also strong involvement of software in the work process to be discussed.

Do not try to save money by having only one person go on a site visit. During the visit you will be talking about complicated, often subtle, process details, and there will be too much going on to expect one person to absorb it all. If travel budget is an issue, as it usually is, it is far better to prioritize and make fewer visits than to try to cover it all and get important details wrong.

*Worst-case.* Site visits are best left until after the questionnaires have been compiled, analyzed, and thoroughly digested. Only then will you know for sure whom you want to visit and why. However, occasionally a worst-case situation arises in which administration of the questionnaire must be combined with the site visit. For example, the project schedule may have slipped because of a key member's absence. If you are considering this combined approach, be sure that it is absolutely necessary and that the issues you wish to cover have been made completely clear. Prepare for the inevitable misses, misunderstanding, and confusion by telling your hosts that they can expect follow-up calls after you have had a chance to digest the results of the visit.

By the time you are ready for a site visit, the broad outlines of the message you wish to convey to your management are beginning to take shape. It is often possible to develop an outline of your project report at this stage, listing the subjects to be covered, and

| PHASE II DATA COLLECTION/ ANALYSIS |
| --- |
| Step 4: Administering Questionnaire |
| Step 5: Analyzing the Data |
| Step 6: Identifying Best Practices |
| Step 7: Doing Site Visits |

agree on assignments for preparation of the various sections of the report. (It is not necessary to draft the report content at this time. See Figure 11 on page 121 of the Blood Bank case study for a sample report outline.)

## SITE VISIT PROTOCOL

PHASE II
DATA
COLLECTION/
ANALYSIS

Step 4:
Administering
Questionnaire

Step 5:
Analyzing the
Data

Step 6:
Identifying
Best Practices

Step 7: Doing
Site Visits

- Make personal contact with the person who will be your host. Agree on:
  - agenda — the purpose of the visit.
  - arrival and departure times.
  - any logistical details (hotel arrangements, maps, transportation, interview rooms, plant tour, etc.).
  - whom you will talk to in probing for greater depth about key subjects revealed by answers to the questionnaire.
  - how the discussions will take place (with individuals or in group session).
    
    **Note:** a group session will often make for a richer and more informative discussion.
  - how and when results will be fed back, providing assurance of confidentiality. (If there has been prior discussion of a reciprocal visit, this is a good time to repeat the offer.)

- If possible, firm up these agreements with a written schedule of events prior to arrival. (Don't be rigid, however — you are a guest, and the host institution is doing you a favor.)

- One visitor should conduct the discussion, listen, and watch the answers (body language!), while the other visitor should record the answers. Trade off roles from time to time.

- As soon as possible after the visit is done, site visitors should caucus privately to agree on what was heard, perhaps even before leaving the site. Sometimes you may want to do this between discussions on the individual topics. Explain to the host that this is only to be sure you got it all straight.

- At the end, behave like a proper departing guest. Repeat the invitation for a reciprocal visit.
- Team members draft assigned portions of the project report as soon as possible after completion of site visit.

## UPDATING FINDINGS AND DRAFT RECOMMENDATIONS

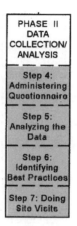

PHASE II
DATA
COLLECTION/
ANALYSIS

Step 4:
Administering
Questionnaire

Step 5:
Analyzing the
Data

Step 6:
Identifying
Best Practices

Step 7: Doing
Site Visits

Following the site visit(s), incorporate the additional information and insights you gathered into the body of your findings. Also, be sure to check whether any of your draft conclusions and action recommendations are altered by the new findings.

You are now ready to approach your sponsor, other stakeholders, and executive-level management to present your findings and begin obtaining concurrence and support for your recommended actions.

### Checklist for a Successful Phase II

- Benchmarking partners given ample support in answering the questionnaire.
- All findings compiled promptly.
- All ambiguities clarified with follow-up calls.
- Annotated findings compilation given to all team members prior to the meeting where they were discussed.
- Team consensus on the findings achieved.
- Best practice descriptions given to all team members prior to the meeting where they were discussed.
- Best practices — and how they work — fully understood.
- Greatest opportunities identified.
- Site visits (if applicable) prepared thoroughly.
- Preliminary drafts of recommended actions prepared.
- Gap profile kept confidential for the present.

## Possible Phase II Pitfalls

### Step 4: Administering the Questionnaire

- Assuming respondents need no support
- Administering a lengthy questionnaire over the telephone
- Administering questionnaire during site visit

### Step 5: Analyzing the Data

- Overanalysis, overprecision
- Wandering from the purpose
- Ambiguous responses not clarified
- Lack of full team consensus on the findings

PHASE II
DATA
COLLECTION/
ANALYSIS

Step 4:
Administering
Questionnaire

Step 5:
Analyzing the
Data

Step 6:
Identifying
Best Practices

Step 7: Doing
Site Visits

### Step 6: Identifying Best Practices

- Not identifying the reasons why best practices are effective
- Not identifying circumstances that enable best practices
- Assumptions not stated when making gap projections
- Overprecision in making gap projections

### Step 7: Doing Site Visits

- Unjustifiable site visits
- Lack of clear understanding of the visit agenda
- Poor logistical preparation for site visits
- One-person site visits

# Chapter 3

# Phase III: Integration

*Phase III begins when a possible set of recommended actions and improvement goals based on the findings begins to emerge, and concludes with the delivery of the benchmarking team's recommendations into the hands of those who will be responsible for turning them into actual work.*

Along the way you will answer a number of key questions:

What is the true purpose of Step 8: Communicating the results?

Why is Step 8 the most difficult?

What is the role of the sponsor at this stage?

Why does Phase III have political aspects?

How do we develop the basis for negotiation with the stakeholders?

How should we approach the various stakeholders — the process owner(s), workforce, administrative staff, and executives?

Why is a neatly bound report not appropriate at this stage?

What is the stylistic difference between Step 8 and Step 9: Establishing goals?

What should we expect to be doing in Step 9?

At the conclusion of Phase III the team will be ready to hand over the lead to the people who will be doing the actual work.

# STEP 8: COMMUNICATING THE RESULTS

The true purpose of Step 8 is **to extend ownership** of the findings and action recommendations beyond the benchmarking team itself. This step is about communication with the sponsor, the stakeholder populations, and with decision-making management. We all communicate on a daily basis, thus one might think that it should require very little attention in a volume like this. However, Step 8 is the trickiest step in the process, and most often done poorly. It requires careful preparation.

It is not hard to understand why Step 8 has great trouble-making possibilities. The benchmarking team has become expert in a particular subject — they see its importance, they have a broadened perspective on where their own institution stands on it, and they *just know* what to do about it. The other folks in the organization don't necessarily share any of this. If they have heard anything at all, it is probably a distorted version of what the benchmarking project is about, what it has done, and how the findings will impact their own work. So communications from the team start off behind the eight-ball, and it is well to plan the next moves keeping this in mind.

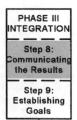

## STRATEGY AND PROCESS

After the site visits, if any, team members should assimilate the additional findings and insights that they have obtained, using the same general approach as in Steps 5 and 6. They should then meet with the sponsor and go over what they have found out, concluding with their (still malleable) ideas for recommended actions.

At this meeting, the sponsor should act as the benchmarking team's customer. Up until now, the sponsor's main function has been to establish and maintain a good working environment, enabling the team to do its best work. His or her next major job is to examine the "product" — the findings and recommended actions — from an evaluative point of view to see how they measure up to expectations.

First, the sponsor should probe the team's methodological rigor, proper use of logic, and breadth of perspective, all in the interests of testing the strength of the case for the action recommendations. If the sponsor has been following the project closely (usually via informal briefings from the team leader), this part of the meeting could go quickly, and you can get right to your proposed actions. However, if for some reason a considerable explanation is necessary to make the sponsor comfortable with the solidity of the findings and the process used to achieve them, the time is well spent.

The outcome of this dialogue should be joint ownership by team and sponsor of the findings of the benchmarking project. That is, both team and sponsor should understand and be ready to advocate the findings.

Next, the sponsor should take up the draft recommendations in a similar kind of dialogue. The end-point of this discussion should be agreement on the recommended actions, again with joint ownership by team and sponsor. In situations where the sponsor is serving as representative of the executive committee, the sponsor should be thinking about how to communicate the recommendations to that body.

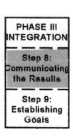

After both team and sponsor have become comfortable with the basis for the team's findings and recommendations, the next job is to extend ownership, particularly of the recommended actions, to as many of the stakeholders as possible. (Remember that a stakeholder is anyone whose work life will be affected by the changes being recommended.) Now you have to decide on what you want to communicate, and to whom.

Here we pass from the realm of "just-the-facts-ma'am" to a world where perceptions count. In our time the word *politics* has come to have some very negative connotations, but by *political* we mean that individuals and groups can have legitimately different perceptions of what constitutes the best thing for the organization as a whole and their own department in particular. These differences in perception mix with the facts, leading inexorably to the need for politically motivated compromises. The old saw that "politics is the art of the possible" captures this point.

The amount of compromise that may be necessary is completely situation-dependent. You may, however, want a few pointers on how to develop a compromise strategy. What follows may seem like pretty elementary stuff, but the whole team must participate in selling your project recommendations, and coming to a consensus on what matters the most and the approach to be used is not always easy.

Working as a team, do the following:

1. Identify the elements of your ideal set of recommended actions — what you would like to see happen in a world without compromise.

2. Identify the elements of your set of recommended actions that are most critical to the success of your organization— without them, the desired improvement (or introduction of the new service) would be severely jeopardized. These you must reserve from compromise if at all possible.

3. Identify the elements of your set of recommended actions that are most likely to arouse resistance, from whom, and why.

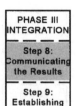

4. Identify the elements that are least critical and/or that are not as strongly supported by your project's findings. These are bargaining chips in case of need.

You have now attached *values* to your tentative set of action recommendations — you know what parts you want most strongly for people to support, and what parts may be compromised away as the price of support.

From here on it is largely a matter of communication. The things to think about in any communication are:

What is the message?

Who is receiving it?

Who is sending it?

What is the vehicle for communication?

What is the process for communication?

Here again we are talking about elementary matters, but remember that everyone on the team must feel that they understand and are comfortable with the game plan for communicating the message.

### The Message

The message you are about to communicate is disruptive: your institution must make some changes in the way it does its business. Most people will not be thrilled to get such a message. Be sure that you have an accurate assessment of which *parts* of your set of recommendations will be seen as most disruptive.

### The Receivers

The changes you are about to propose will have different impacts on different stakeholders. Some groups may be affected only peripherally. Others will be seriously shaken up, but if you carried out Step 1 conscientiously they will be well represented on the benchmarking team. The representatives of the most seriously disrupted groups should be able to gauge the level of receptiveness to be expected from their colleagues and have useful ideas about how to approach them, both individually and collectively, with the message. Practically speaking, informal progress-reporting by these representatives in the form of answers to the "How's it going?" type of question will by this time probably have allowed the broad outlines of what is in store to become known to key people, and their basic reactions to be noted.

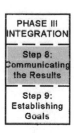

PHASE III
INTEGRATION

Step 8:
Communicating
the Results

Step 9:
Establishing
Goals

### The Senders

Your benchmarking team is a well-balanced group of experienced and responsible members of the organization. The team was put together with representatives from the groups that will be most affected by the message, and presumably with their full backing. It does well to remind these groups that what they are about to hear comes from people they know and trust. It also does well for the team members to remind themselves that the stakeholders they will be talking to are also, in a very real sense, customers for their findings and recommendations.

## The Vehicle

The surest way to call forth resistance to change is to announce it abruptly on a "take it or leave it" basis. And yet this is inevitably the impression created by a neatly bound, signed-off-by-management benchmarking team report when it is received in the mail by someone who will be required to implement its recommendations. Never leave people without recourse.

A simple way around this recipe for disaster is to go with your recommendations *while they are still in draft form* to get the reaction of individuals and groups who will be heavily impacted by them. Sometimes you will be surprised at how easily major changes are accepted if small (to you) modifications are made in the way they are presented. At other times, a fundamentally better way to achieve the work process improvement objective may emerge from these discussions. If feasible changes that do not compromise your recommendations are proposed for whatever reason by the people who have to do the work, make the changes. It helps to extend ownership.

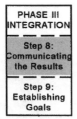

Another way to extend ownership of your ideas is to share credit for their creation. Those who find this hard to do should ask themselves: "Which do I want most, the credit for stating the idea or the satisfaction of seeing the idea in action?"

Sometimes it will be necessary to override objections. When this happens your case is always strengthened if the objectors agree that their objections have been heard, understood, considered, and set aside for reasons that have been explained to them.

## The Communication Process

Local culture and custom will always dictate the communication process. Simply remember that your object is to *extend ownership* of your conclusions and recommendations, and certain individuals and groups either must or should be enlisted. One approach is as follows:

- *The Process Owner(s).* The **process owner** is the person in management responsible and accountable for the service or product that is to be improved or introduced. If there is only one process owner, the battle is half over, because he or she is already represented on the benchmarking team, has been kept up to date on the activities of the team, and feels considerable ownership already. In this case, you request an appointment, prepare a summary of your methodology, your findings, and your proposed recommendations (prominently marked "draft"), send them to the individual in question, and go to the meeting prepared to answer questions. Even if s/he did not read the material you submitted prior to the meeting, its presence will help to focus the discussion.

When talking about the methodology and findings, be as crisp and brief as possible, consistent with achieving a high comfort index and answering the questions. But when you get to the recommendations, slow down and be as receptive to other viewpoints as possible. Know what you can agree to on the spot and what will require team consideration. (Here is where having team agreement on when you can compromise pays off.)

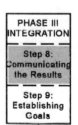

Leave with as clear a statement as possible about the process owner's level of support for your recommendations.

More often than not, however, particularly if we are talking about a new service, several departments may be affected by your proposed actions. There will be several interacting processes, and several process owners. Here you can go either of two ways — try to get a group meeting with all the affected individuals, or tackle them one at a time.

As a practical matter, it is usually much easier to schedule several one-on-one sessions than a group discussion. There are other advantages as well, such as the fact that not everyone will be equally interested in the same topics, and you can tailor your emphasis to one person at a time. Be sure, however, that you tell the same story to everyone. Emphasis is one thing, but content is something else!

Again, get a clear a statement of support for your recommendations, noting any differences among the people you have contacted.

- *The Workforce.* What you desire is fresh, independent, knowledgeable, respected, and discreet reactions to the changes you intend to propose. It is impossible to generalize on how to do this. We suggest bringing a few "guest experts" in for key discussions of the benchmarking team. This helps to keep the team from coming to inappropriate conclusions for whatever reason. Sometimes a quiet, private discussion is indicated. Sometimes it is best not to do anything at all. However, it is very persuasive to say that you have tried out your ideas on so-and-so, and she likes them. ("So-and-so" being a widely known and respected old hand — every organization has them.)

- *The Administrative Staff.* Here we are talking about the support people who prepare budgets, human resources, facilities, and the like. If your recommendations will include significant changes in spending, staffing, materials acquisition, space, plant engineering, or other similar activities, it is well worth the effort to get the reaction of the people who do this kind of work. Simply catching the budget preparation cycle at the right time is often an enormous help in getting a big initiative off to a good start.

- *The Executive Committee.* This group should be the last on your schedule. At this stage you should be able to say that you have support from the process owner(s), the workers, the support functions, and that your needs are understood and supported by the administrative staff. In short, the feasibility and acceptability of the action plan is established. The executive group is thus free to concentrate on the policy and financial priorities of your proposals.

PHASE III
INTEGRATION

Step 8:
Communicating
the Results

Step 9:
Establishing
Goals

If your benchmarking project has sufficient scope and importance, it may be necessary to gain the support of this group as a whole. Often it is sufficient to go to the one member of the executive body who has overall responsibility in the area where your project lies. For example, a project addressing the upgrade of laboratory instrumentation, which would probably be sponsored by the laboratory's director, may need executive-level support by the medical director and CFO and no others, whereas a project to change the entire organization's information system would definitely require full Executive Committee concurrence. In either case, contact at this level is best left to the team sponsor.

It is at this stage that the value of high-level sponsorship of the benchmarking project is recognized. Such a sponsor can keep peers apprised of progress in the project quite easily and relatively informally, so that when the recommendations come up for their review and concurrence, it is not as if a foreign object had fallen from the sky. In the Stroke Therapy Initiative case, for example, the sponsor kept his peers up to date, and at their own request.

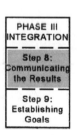

## Content

So far we have talked about the strategy and process for your communications. Now let's talk in more detail about the substance of what you plan to communicate. A benchmarking project follows a **methodology** and produces two kinds of results: **findings** and **recommendations** based on the findings.

*Methodology.* Yours is a potentially shocking message, and you had better convince your audience(s) that you know what you are talking about. One of the most important aspects of your findings is the methodology, or the protocol, you used to produce them (a point very familiar to people in healthcare). Methodology must be clear, preferably documented, and above all, followed. Documentation need not be elaborate. Brief minutes of meetings, with attached copies of homework materials circulated prior to meetings is usually enough. Full transcription of the ubiquitous flip-charts can usually be avoided if done carefully.

Feel free to communicate the methodology (but *not* the findings) at any time to anyone who wishes to know, even if only out of curiosity. You can't have too many friends.

*Findings and recommendations.* These must be communicated together as a unified message. Never go to anyone, no matter how informally, with unsupported recommendations.

*Findings.* Your findings, the what and how, are the basis for your recommendations, and should lead your audience to the same appraisal of the situation that you made. One good way to do this is to organize your key "what" results into a table comparing your performance and that of your benchmarking partners, as in the Blood Bank case. If you do this, be sure that this table is not cluttered with interesting (to you) details that draw attention away from the main message. Keep to the main points.

You also want to stimulate your audience to ask spontaneously: "What do you think we should do about this situation you have described?"

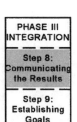

Their mind-set will now be action-oriented and more receptive to ideas about new ways of doing things. You should then be ready with the other half of your story: the things you learned about *how* your benchmarking partners achieve their superior performance. Again, keep it focused on key findings that lead persuasively to the recommendations.

*Recommendations.* What kinds of recommendations come out of a benchmarking project? Recalling that the project was chartered to address an overall objective, it should come as no surprise that the project should produce recommendations about what should be done to achieve the objective, and how to do it.

In the Blood Bank case, where the overall objective is to improve the operation of the blood bank, the team said:

"Reduce delivery delays to the OPD (what should be done) by adopting/adapting the Western Medical Center practice of placing routine orders in advance (how to do it)."

In the Ischemic Stroke Initiative case, the overall objective of the benchmarking project part of the program was to convince everyone involved that a stroke is a true emergency. The team said:

"Be sure that everyone who will be affected by or involved in carrying out the ISI is given at least as much information as they will need to perform their function (what should be done). All members of every group involved in carrying out the new stroke protocol should be provided with the same basic package of information (how to do it)."

What to do and how to do it, nothing else. There is a danger at this point in the project, arising from the broadened perspective and heightened awareness that the team has acquired by looking at the outside world. There is an understandable temptation to stray beyond the boundaries of the charter, and offer suggestions about some of the other problems and deficiencies that have come to the team's attention, however peripherally. Don't let it happen. Stick to your subject or you will suffer erosion of your credibility and the desertion of your supporters.

What you want is a **consensus** in support of your recommendations. The Japanese, who have raised consensus-building to the level of an art form, have given us an operational definition of consensus that should be your guide in discussing your proposed recommendations with anyone whose support you solicit. In the Japanese operational definition, each party to a consensus can say:

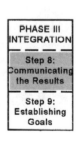

- "I have heard what you have to say."

- "You have heard what I have to say."

- "Whereas we may not agree totally on everything, we each agree to support the proposal in its present form".

Clearly this recipe for getting everyone behind your recommended approach requires some forthright give and take. The people whose support you are seeking will sense whether you are genuinely receptive to their thoughts or just going through the motions. This is why it is a good idea to think of your recommendations as a *draft* for consideration by your intended supporters, even if it is the most carefully crafted set of statements that you can produce. With this mind-set and a clear picture of the overall objective, negotiation with the stakeholders is on-course to a good outcome.

Many books have been written about the mechanics of communication, and it would serve you well to study and keep their lessons in mind, but if you remember that the purpose of Step 8 is to *extend ownership* of your action plan, you will not go seriously wrong.

# STEP 9: ESTABLISHING GOALS

In Step 8, the goal was to reach an agreement in principle on what to do and how to do it. Step 9 becomes quantitative: it addresses the questions of how much, how far, how fast, and by whom. In other words, assignments can now be given to specific groups and individuals to make measurable progress toward measurable goals.

In a sense, Step 9 is a replay of Step 8 with an additional level of detail. In Step 8 we proceeded from acceptance of the overall objective to agreement on what to do and how to do it in order to achieve that objective. In Step 9, we proceed from ownership extension of the actions to be taken to agreement on more detailed statements about these actions and measures of success for carrying them out.

PHASE III
INTEGRATION

Step 8:
Communicating
the Results

Step 9:
Establishing
Goals

## COMPLETING OWNERSHIP TRANSFER

It should come as no surprise that the most effective way to set achievable goals is to involve those who will have to deliver the results in the establishment of these goals. However, instead of the *persuasion* that characterized Step 8, the approach in Step 9 is essentially a *teaching* function.

Specifically, the groups responsible for making it all happen must fully understand both the power and the problems involved with the new approaches. Only when they feel comfortable with their ability to practice the new work processes will they be able to gauge what they will be able to accomplish using them, and how long it will take to do so. To put it bluntly, if the implementers are to *own their goals*, they have to know what they are getting into. It is the job of the benchmarking team to transfer as much detailed knowledge as possible to the people who will do the work.

As with other forms of communication, whole libraries have been written about teaching, much of it applicable to the benchmarking process. However, there are a few aspects of Step 9 that deserve specific mention.

- Evaluate the size of the teaching task. If the benchmarking project has a narrow focus, teaching may come down to a few people sitting down and going over the findings together. Some projects, on the other hand, will involve so many different groups in implementing the new and/or improved process that formal instructional materials may have to be prepared. For example, in the Stroke Therapy Initiative case, the whole action plan was, to a large extent, one giant teaching job.

- Remember what you want from your teaching. The end result of Step 9 is a set of goals established by the same people who will become accountable for them. They must be satisfied that the goals are achievable, and they must be motivated enough to achieve them. Keep the discussion focused on what you know about the effectiveness of the new/improved processes and what is required to make them work well.

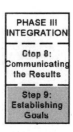

  Here is where a well-chosen team roster really pays off. Among professional people, knowledgeable discussion of the nitty-gritty details of a process modification, led by someone from their own specialty whom they know either personally or by reputation, is far more compelling than all the glittering generalities of someone brought in from elsewhere.

- Remember that you are carrying out a brokering task as well: management will have some ideas about how far and how fast things should proceed, and the people who will have to make it happen may develop other, more cautious ideas. Somehow these differing viewpoints must be brought into harmony, and that is part of the job of the benchmarking team. One very effective way to set the stage for this is to have the team sponsor explain management's view of the importance of the work ahead, and their high hopes for successful progress. It sometimes happens, however, that the implementers without any prompting, will set stretch goals that management would never dare to think of. As usual, it is situational.

Many people feel the completion of Phase III marks the end of the benchmarking team's job. You have delivered your recommendations into the hands of those who will be responsible for turning them into actual work.

Except for a final report (which can be very modest in length because its main purposes have been accomplished as you went along), you may be done. Metaphorically, the synapse between the nervous system (management) and the muscle (work force) has been made.

However, the team, or a few key members, may be asked to participate in Phase IV. As illustrated in the next chapter, this is usually a good idea, and we will proceed on that assumption.

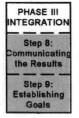

## Checklist for a Successful Phase III

- Ownership of the findings and recommendations by the team's first customer — the team sponsor — established.
- Elements of the recommended actions evaluated and a strategy for compromise developed.
- Feedback on the draft recommendations obtained from the process owner(s)
- Project methodology, findings, and recommendations organized, in that order.
- Team consensus established on the content of the message, how to deliver it, and to what audiences.

- Stakeholders' ideas and suggestions acknowledged, and used where feasible.
- The team's role as teacher understood and carried out.

## Possible Phase III Pitfalls

### Step 8: Communicating the Results

- Parading your newfound expertise
- Hogging all the credit
- Going with unsupported recommendations
- Leaving people with no recourse — recommendations cast in concrete
- Wandering off into interesting by-paths

### Step 9: Establishing Goals

- Neglecting the responsibility to teach
- Not letting go gracefully when asked
- Prematurely abandoning interest in the planning

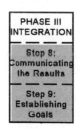

PHASE III
INTEGRATION

Step 8:
Communicating
the Results

Step 9:
Establishing
Goals

# Chapter 4

# Phase IV: Action

*In Phase IV, the benchmarking process goes public, and a whole new set of dynamics manifests itself, with the importance of continuity becoming apparent.*

It might be a good idea at this point to remind ourselves of some basic ideas. Benchmarking is one integrated process consisting of several subprocesses or phases. All of these subprocesses — Planning, Data Collection and Analysis, Integration, and Action — are things we all do regularly. As pointed out in the Introduction, when practiced individually, they provide nothing new. Consider:

*Planning.* When done for its own sake, the output of planning is a report, which usually gathers dust in credenzas and libraries.

*Data Collection and Analysis.* When done for their own sake, the output is again a report or its equivalent, which few understand and no one acts upon. All by themselves, data collection and analysis won't change the world.

*Integration.* When done in isolation, arguing for the integration of a new idea or approach into the organization's goals and objectives degenerates into a game of intellectual arm-wrestling in which we find out whose ideas will prevail, not which ideas are the best.

*Action.* There is an old saying: "Nothing is as frightening as ignorance in action." And yet that is exactly what you will most likely get if you leap into action without going through the preceding phases.

The power of benchmarking stems from the fact that these well-known activities are assembled into an *integrated process* with a single overall purpose: to improve the organization's performance.

This power is dissipated and lost if the thread leading from Phase III to Phase IV is broken. It is critical that the integration — the continuity with what has been done so far — be preserved. It is a truism that *only the people who do the work know how the work* **really** *gets done*. A corollary of this is that if the people who do the work are not persuaded of the benefits of a new approach, it won't be long before the new approach becomes an orphan.

Thus, our focus in Phase IV will be on ensuring that the knowledge gained is not lost and that there is no change in intent or intensity as responsibility is passed from the benchmarking team to the process team. We want to ensure that action is based on the planning, data collection, analysis, and integration with the organization's goals and objectives carried out in the preceding three phases and takes full advantage of what has been learned during the benchmarking project.

Along the way you will answer a number of key questions:

> How can we be sure that the knowledge and insights gained so far are not lost in the hand-off?
>
> Should the benchmarking team bow out at this point?
>
> Why should a member of the benchmarking team stay on?
>
> How does it feel to be an innocent victim of unannounced change?

At the conclusion of Phase IV your organization should be measuring and beginning to enjoy the benefits of taking informed action using the best available methods to achieve the original objective.

PHASE IV
ACTION

Step 10:
Developing
Action Plans

Step 11:
Implementing
the Plan/
Monitoring
Results

Step 12:
Revisiting the
Subject

## STEP 10: DEVELOPING ACTION PLANS

Put yourself in the frame of mind of a parent watching a maturing child leave home — you know your son or daughter is not quite ready, but you have to let go eventually and it might as well be now. That is how a benchmarking project team usually feels at this point.

The team's work is done, really, and the hand-off must be made, but you wish you could be sure the receivers won't drop the ball.

Why do you feel that way?

- You now know things about doing the work that were not known before in your organization — you wouldn't have gone a-benchmarking if this were not the case.

- You didn't write it all down — impossible and unnecessary — but you know that a lot of that untransmitted detail is very important to making a good plan and carrying it out successfully.

- You have developed lines of communication, both at management and working levels, which can make it a lot easier to get things to happen — you have influential contacts, and you can smooth the way.

- But you also know that the people who are accountable must do the work, and they must do two things that you can't do for them: become filled with the desire to make it work (take ownership), and make the detailed adaptations of what you found out to the local working environment (develop the action plan).

All these feelings are legitimate. So what should the benchmarking team therefore do? There are two ways the team can play a significant role at this point: help with the planning and help with organizationwide communication.

## PLANNING

Many healthcare organizations have a lot of trouble with formal planning. The reasons for this are obscure to us, but in our experience, the practice of preparing a yearly operating plan, with goals, mileposts, budgets, and progressively more detailed work assignments — the whole paraphernalia of planning that is taken for granted in industry — is largely confined to the Finance Department. In most operating departments, particularly the clinical departments, planning usually has a very short time horizon. If

| PHASE IV ACTION |
|---|
| Step 10: Developing Action Plans |
| Step 11: Implementing the Plan/ Monitoring Results |
| Step 12: Revisiting the Subject |

your institution does not traditionally implement forward planning at the level of the people responsible for the important details of the work processes, and a good plan is necessary to ensure the success of a major change, help in preparing the plan must be supplied.

---

## PLANNING MYOPIA

People tend to apply to their professional activities what E. L. Doctorow is said to have remarked about writing a novel: "It's like an automobile trip by night — your headlights can only illuminate the road for the next few hundred yards, but that doesn't stop you from making a trip of a few hundred miles."

There is enough truth in this aphorism as it applies to small changes in well-known work activities that a lot of individuals and organizations have been able to get by for decades by not extending their horizon beyond the boundaries of their own department and its activities for the next several weeks. However, in times of rapid change, this approach practically guarantees crisis management, and fosters the "silo mentality" rightly deplored by systems thinkers as the enemy of healthy organizations.

Moreover, it just won't work *whenever* large changes are to be made in work processes that involve a number of stakeholding groups.

---

**PHASE IV ACTION**

**Step 10:** Developing Action Plans

**Step 11:** Implementing the Plan/ Monitoring Results

**Step 12:** Revisiting the Subject

Much of this help can come from the financial planning staff. In Step 8 the benchmarking team was counseled to inform finance people (as well as other administrative functions) about its findings and recommendations. Now is the time to get them actively involved in supporting the process owner(s) and their professional specialists in planning the contemplated changes. If no individual or group in administration has the responsibility for preparing, or managing the preparation of, operating plans for the organization, the benchmarking team may volunteer to help get the detailed plans put together. If there is a group responsible for planning, the team still should be available to help, but in a somewhat different capacity. (See the third appendix for a short discussion of the practicalities of successful planning at this stage.)

Recalling that at this juncture a balance must be struck between letting go and being there when needed, probably the best thing for the benchmarking team to do is to dismantle its ability to *do* the planning, while keeping the ability to offer *good advice*. Accordingly, successful benchmarking project teams generally discontinue organized activity at this juncture, being sure that someone is appointed *in loco parentis*, as it were. This person can answer the telephone, see what needs to be provided that may have been overlooked, clarify obscure points from the findings, and generally *smooth* the way without getting *in* the way.

The best person(s) for this job is usually the representative on the benchmarking team from the department(s) where the largest work process change(s) will take place; often this will be the team leader. Sometimes it will be a team member with unusually good people skills—for example, Mr. Sam Adams in the St. Luke's Hospital Information System Changeover case study. Regardless of who he or she may be, the holdover team member should be assured of instant access to the team leader, the sponsor, and other team members as needed.

The output of Step 10 is the detailed action plan for implementing the recommended changes. If the benchmarking team or a holdover member is asked to review the plan, these are the things to watch for:

- A clear statement of the plan's objective.
- A timeline with defined intermediate goals at specific points.
- Defined measurements for deciding whether or not the intermediate goals were achieved.
- Financial resources required to achieve the goals, preferably with a time profile of usage.

| PHASE IV ACTION |
| --- |
| Step 10: Developing Action Plans |
| Step 11: Implementing the Plan/ Monitoring Results |
| Step 12: Revisiting the Subject |

- Staffing required, preferably with names and a time profile of assignments.

- Space, equipment, and general support services required.

- Provision for a small-scale tryout of the new or improved service in a pilot implementation, if appropriate.

## COMMUNICATION

Most healthcare organizations do a good job of communication. From the daily shift-change briefings to the innumerable clinical consults to the organization's weekly news-sheet to formal state-of-the-institution presentations by upper management, there are plenty of official avenues for communication, not to mention the vigorous grapevine where most of the real dope is purveyed, to many people's way of thinking. So there should be no communications issue to address, right? Wrong.

Don't forget that the usual channels of communication were purposely limited for a time during the benchmarking project, and this more than likely led to a virulent spread of rumors when inklings of what was going on inevitably escaped. Imagine what it must be like in this era of downsizing, job description instability, and general chaos to learn through the rumor mill that your function is being completely "reengineered," whatever that may mean to you. As recently as 10 years ago it was almost impossible for anyone in high-level management to imagine the emotions of people in the lower reaches of the organizational hierarchy when a major reorganization was rumored. But nowadays no one is unacquainted with these feelings, and empathy is that much easier to experience. But it must be acted upon.

So the first task in taking the project public is to put out a complete story of the situation in an institutionwide publication. The story should tell why the project was undertaken, the overall objective, who was involved, who will be affected, how the work was done, what the findings were, what decisions were made, what the consequences will be, when they will be felt, and by whom.

Note that coverage should be complete, but no more *detailed* than appropriate. It is more important for people to get an undis-

PHASE IV
ACTION

Step 10:
Developing
Action Plans

Step 11:
Implementing
the Plan/
Monitoring
Results

Step 12:
Revisiting the
Subject

torted overview than a bunch of details that tend to obscure the main message. Also, confidentiality in some areas may need to be preserved.

This comprehensive summary should be circulated widely and as soon as possible. You will want to leave plenty of time for the facts to percolate through the organization. For one thing, the skeptics, who are in abundant supply and potentially your best friends, need to get the facts and chew on them in order to turn themselves around. Don't forget that the skeptics have plenty of basis for their skepticism: every organization has made its little missteps to feed the flames. Also, the cynics need to be marginalized, and the best way to refute corrosive rumors is with honest facts. The benchmarking team itself, or the holdover representative, can help prepare this communication to the rest of the workforce, assisting whoever has the responsibility for putting out the news in your organization.

Finally, a few useful behaviors for the Step 10 team holdover person:

- Don't hover. Give the people with operational responsibility plenty of room to find things out for themselves. But stand ready to fill in gaps in their information — the stuff that never got written down.

- Be ready to move fast when necessary. Inevitably, something will get left out that has to be provided in a hurry. An example from the St. Luke's Information System Changeover case study is the need to bring a vendor representative out on short notice to deal with an unforeseen software problem. Here's where your greater visibility and influential contacts can pay off handsomely.

- Be the conscience of the planning process. Be sure that the original intent is properly addressed, that the original goals are not watered down, and that measurements are put in place to keep track of performance during implementation.

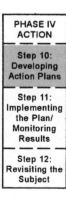

PHASE IV
ACTION

Step 10:
Developing
Action Plans

Step 11:
Implementing
the Plan/
Monitoring
Results

Step 12:
Revisiting the
Subject

## STEP 11: IMPLEMENTING THE PLAN/ MONITORING RESULTS

In Step 10, measurements to help in monitoring process performance and output quality were identified. Management at both the operational and executive level may ask the benchmarking team to review the results of these measurements from time to time. Do so if asked, but only then. Remember, the overall objective is to improve the performance of your institution, and the only people who can do that now are the people who do the work and are accountable for the results. Nothing the benchmarking team does should diminish these people's feelings of ownership and accountability.

However, you are now very knowledgeable about the benchmarking process. Watching the detailed implementation effort will give insights into what could have been done better to make the project and the passing of the baton go better. In the spirit of continuous improvement, you will want to identify the **lessons learned** and write them down. Representative examples of lessons learned can be found in the Epilogue to the Information System Changeover case study.

Now is also the time to recognize and reward the benchmarking team for its efforts. Part of this is celebration of your success. Another part is a thoughtfully prepared evaluation of each team member's contribution. In the discussion of team recruiting in Step 1 it was pointed out that participation in a benchmarking team should be a *formal objective* for team members, perhaps displacing other objectives if the project is a very large one. An objective review should be carried out for each team member and for any guest experts who did a significant amount of work, with appropriate reward for outstanding performance. These actions are a joint responsibility of the team leader and the sponsor working together. The objective review is particularly important for the longer term, because it will strongly influence whether potential members of any future benchmarking projects will dare risk volunteering when the time comes.

PHASE IV
ACTION

Step 10:
Developing
Action Plans

Step 11:
Implementing
the Plan/
Monitoring
Results

Step 12:
Revisiting the
Subject

# STEP 12: REVISITING THE SUBJECT

One of the axioms of Continuous Quality Improvement is that every process and every output is capable of being improved without limit. However, this is not to say that everything has equal priority. It is foolish to add one more decimal point to one measurement while another important dimension goes completely unquantified. As the old Vermonter said: "Only a waste-thrift would plane the underside of a privy seat."

So when a benchmarking project is put to bed, it does well to include in the final recommendations a statement about the circumstances under which it will be appropriate to revisit the subject you addressed. Sometimes you will simply want to note that the area should be revisited in perhaps 2 years. In other cases a more elaborate recommendation based on relative performance, or rate of performance improvement may become the criterion.

### Checklist for a Successful Phase IV

- Project relinquished to the accountable process team.
- One team member designated as a contact to help in planning.
- Implementation plan reviewed for completeness and clarity.
- Procedure for monitoring progress in implementing the plan ensured.
- A lessons-learned document for future benchmarking teams developed.
- Completion of the project celebrated.
- Objective reviews and concomitant rewards prepared for project participants.
- Criteria for revisiting the subject identified.

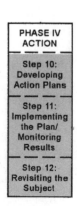

## Possible Phase IV Pitfalls

### Step 10: Developing Action Plans

- Smothering the process team with attention
- Being unavailable when needed

### Step 11: Implementing the Plan/Monitoring Results

- Allowing unquantifiable intermediate goals into the plan
- Not recognizing the work of the benchmarking team
- Not reviewing and rewarding appropriately the performance of benchmarking team members individually

### Step 12: Revisiting the Subject

- Leaving vague instructions about when to revisit the subject

PHASE IV
ACTION

Step 10:
Developing
Action Plans

Step 11:
Implementing
the Plan/
Monitoring
Results

Step 12:
Revisiting the
Subject

# Part II
# Case Studies

## OVERVIEW

Part II is in the form of four fictitious case studies. Each case study is told in short-story format, with the key project documents and process descriptions included as easily referenced exhibits.

- **Chapter 5: Benchmarking Team Perspective. The Blood Bank at Good Samaritan Hospital.** This study addresses operational problems at a blood bank in a large teaching hospital. It is seen from the point of view of the benchmarking team, and includes much detail about what the team actually does. Readers will learn by example such practical things as what the role of the team leader is, how to make their meeting time most effective, what a good benchmarking partner questionnaire looks like, etc.

- **Chapter 6: Sponsor Perspective. Mercy Hospital Stroke Therapy Initiative.** This case study shows how a benchmarking project is used by its sponsor, the person in management for whom the project is done, to avoid unnecessary missteps and delays in implementing a major new emergency medicine protocol, namely, the use of tissue plasminogen activator in treatment of ischemic stroke. The reader will learn, among other things, how to charter and provide support to a benchmarking team, how to keep it on track, and how to use its findings as part of a larger effort.

- **Chapter 7: Top Management Perspective. The Cranbrook Health System's Modernization Crisis.** This study looks at benchmarking activity from the point of view of the Chief Executive Officer of a Health Maintenance Organization. His task is to marshall his management team to solve serious operational problems brought on by an outdated information system in an environment where the HMO may be swallowed up or driven out of business. The central message of this case study is that benchmarking is a tool to help members of upper management focus on things they must do in any event. Examples of use of the benchmarking tool include: how to make good use of board members, how to mentor direct report managers, and how to organize an executive committee strategy discussion for maximum productivity.

- **Chapter 8: Workforce Perspective. Variations on a Theme: St. Luke's Hospital Information System Changeover.** This study describes the changeover to a new internally networked information system, as seen by stakeholders in the workforce. These are people who were not members of the benchmarking team, but whose work lives are changed by the outcome of the benchmarking project. Readers will become sensitized to the impact on the front-line workforce during the startup transient of the new system, seeing some upheavals in the work lives of five typical workers in different functions, how these upheavals can be handled, and how they might have been prevented.

As mentioned in the Introduction, each case study is kept relatively short, concentrating on the actions of a particular category of player, and simply sketching the activities of the other role categories.

Fictionalizing the case studies has freed them from certain constraints, making it possible to show the way benchmarking projects really happen — some rough, some smooth. Seeing how common problems can arise in a realistic story context illustrates for the reader how the warning signs of trouble ahead are likely to manifest themselves in practice, and complements the "Possible Pitfalls" lists found in Chapters 1–4.

Nonetheless, many readers may feel that the stories are still somewhat idealized — in real life, nothing goes quite this smoothly. For example, there is only one instance (in the fourth case study) where an individual's personal behavior steps out of bounds, and yet we all know that the stresses of healthcare work, including the pressures of time and fatigue, frequently push people into uncharacteristically poor behavior. We assume, however, that readers can supply these bits of color themselves. In a certain sense, "when you've seen one temper tantrum, you've seen 'em all." That is, very little can be learned from an ongoing parade of descriptions of abrasive interactions, however much it might add to the realism.

Much more significantly, on the other hand, is that the roles in the case studies are almost all filled by someone *fully qualified to do the job*. There are only two clear-cut examples, one each in the third and fourth case studies, where an individual is simply not up to the task, and bad things happen because of this. In real life, on the other hand, assignments that carry more responsibility than authority or ability to perform happen far more frequently than we would wish.

For example, in the case studies, people call meetings, and the other people all dutifully come to the meetings. This is fine if you are the head of the department or the CEO, and all the people at the meeting work for you, but what if you call a meeting of peers from other organizations, and they are all (legitimately) very busy and some don't show up? In the case studies, a world has been set up where problems of this sort don't happen. In real life, when these problems *do* happen, fall-back positions and "workarounds" must obviously be prepared. These are almost always situational, and the best general preparation is to be on the watch for the signs of trouble. The practical lesson is simply:

> *If you are asked to do a benchmarking job that requires more clout than you normally wield, try to ensure that, along with the delegated responsibility to perform, an appropriate level of authority is provided for your use as well. If this does not hap-*

*pen, you must modify the process you use to make it consistent with the limitations of your real situation.*

One final point. Each of the case studies deals with a real need to learn a better way to do something — improve a blood bank service, roll out a new or upgraded computer system, etc. However, you should not expect to find the answer to *your* specific combination of needs and circumstances in these studies. Enough detail is provided to illustrate realistically the subjects, the sequence, and the processes involved in a benchmarking project, but a one-size-fits-all recipe for fixing tough operational problems is misleading, dangerous, and perhaps even fraudulent. In the Stroke Therapy Initiative case in Chapter 6, for example, it would be ludicrous and offensive to suggest that a complete cost-benefit analysis for anything as complex as a whole new clinical pathway can be compressed into a two-page addendum. What you *can* expect is that the cost-benefit analysis is treated realistically and in sufficient detail to make clear what some of the issues are that must be addressed.

# Chapter 5

# The Blood Bank at Good Samaritan Hospital

## Benchmarking Team Perspective

*The benchmarking team is the group of people responsible for carrying out the benchmarking project. It includes a team leader (usually a person with management experience) and five to eight team members who collectively possess knowledge of the subject and represent all the major stakeholders.*

This case study is about a blood bank that used benchmarking to solve a number of serious operational problems relating to the delivery of blood products. It involves participation by the blood bank and its customers, plus a representative from the organization responsible for transportation of the blood products to the users. The benchmarking project focused on two areas: **what** constitutes superior performance in the operation of a blood bank, and **how** blood banks with superior performance achieved their good results.

Things to watch for in this case study are:

Why and how the team leader gets a benchmarking project started.

How the team charter is used in communicating with the team sponsor.

What to do to ensure that team meeting time is used effectively.

How to use a set of benchmarking project success criteria.

What good meeting minutes look like.

How to use a screener questionnaire to select the most useful benchmarking partners.

What a good set of operational performance metrics looks like.

The structure and administration of a benchmarking partner's questionnaire.

How to prepare for and conduct a site visit.

How to get from project findings to a workable set of recommendations accepted by all the stakeholders.

## THE SITUATION

Good Samaritan is a large (750-bed) hospital serving a 1.5 million catchment population, which is also served by 10 other competing hospitals. It is a teaching hospital, delivering mostly acute care, and has a very active emergency department. About a year ago, Good Samaritan entered into a managed care arrangement with two large HMOs with a combined population of 300,000 subscribers, comprising employees of several major companies in the community, a large number of workers in smaller firms, plus a good-sized population of individual subscribers.

Good Samaritan also began a CQI movement about a year ago, and all employees have participated in a four-hour discussion of what CQI is and what it is expected to do for the hospital. All supervisors and some front-line employees have received two days of training in the tools and techniques of CQI. The hospital administrator has shown by his actions a solid commitment to CQI, but no major benefits have resulted from its introduction so far.

# The Blood Bank at Good Samaritan Hospital

Hit by reimbursement reductions, Good Samaritan is engaged in across-the-board downsizing and cost-reduction actions, including a hiring freeze.

The hospital is currently in the early stages of a cost-of-care study that is being carried out department by department. It began with general support services such as housekeeping, and will soon be moving into clinical support functions.

The Good Samaritan hospital blood bank is staffed by a hardworking and conscientious group of 45 skilled technicians. However, its reputation for reliable service has not been good in recent years, and the blood bank has been having even more trouble than usual recently with delivery of blood products. ("Delivery" is shorthand for the entire work flow from receipt of physician order in the blood bank to start of the patient transfusion.) As a consequence, relations with users are not the best.

The possible reasons for this deterioration in the quality of its services and user relations have been a source of some disagreement among blood bank staff. A few people are convinced that the pneumatic tube system and the back-up messenger service are not functioning properly. Others believe the difficulties are internal to the blood bank. There are also some who blame the users and/or their support staff: floor nurses, nursing unit desk secretaries, surgeons, scrub nurses, and operating room desk personnel.

Last week, the blood bank supervisor, Julie Jones, was informed that her department would be asked to perform a cost study in the near future.

The timing of this request was very inconvenient for the blood bank because Good Samaritan had recently instituted a liver transplant program that had produced some disruptive fluctuations in demand on its blood bank. Also, a new procedure for leucocyte filtration is being inaugurated, with the attendant confusion surrounding any major new process.

Ms. Jones recognized the necessity for preparing her group for the cost study. Because she is a convert to CQI, she decided to approach it in a team spirit with her supervisors, and called a special meeting of her supervisory staff.

| PHASE I<br>PLANNING |
| --- |
| Step 1:<br>Organizing<br>the Project |
| Step 2:<br>Identifying Best<br>Practitioners |
| Step 3:<br>Preparing to<br>Collect Data |

# THE STORY

At the special supervisors' meeting, Ms. Jones announced the impending cost study. She acknowledged the difficult timing with the new programs, and the background of chronic delivery problems. She asked for ideas on how to cope. Alberta Harrington, the dayshift supervisor, suggested a benchmarking project and was immediately challenged by one of her peers: "Why benchmarking? Why not a problem-solving project instead?"

Ms. Harrington agreed that problem-solving is certainly a possibility, that they both require fact-finding and objectivity, and, properly handled, both excite the active interest of all stakeholding groups. However, she said, by its very nature, benchmarking **guarantees entirely fresh thinking** because it requires investigation of how other people deal with the same problems.

In the ensuing discussion, a flood of questions came forth:

- What subject? What scope?
- Who will do it?
- How much work is involved?
- How long will it take?
- Can we get support, or even permission? Can it be done on hospital time?
- Who fills in for people working on the project?
- How do we keep resentment from developing among those not participating in the project?

It soon became clear that these questions were legitimate and that they must be answered. The group decided that they needed a draft project proposal for study, and Alberta volunteered to prepare it for discussion at a meeting to be held in two weeks. At the next meeting, the key elements of Alberta's proposal (Figure 1) were discussed.

- Proposed subject: the blood components delivery process from end to end.
- Team members: five to six people, representatives of all stakeholding operations; plus expert consultation.

- Time: one-half day/week for 3–4 months.
- Resources: overtime for staff filling in for team.
- Communications: THE key to success. All stakeholders must become convinced that the project is being done right, that the right answers will be obtained, and that the right recommendations will be made.
- Travel: site visits planned only after needs for specific process information have been identified.

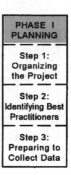

After some discussion of other possible subjects (transplant programs, leucocyte filtration, blood bank costs), the proposal was accepted. It was generally agreed that Alberta had done a great job on the proposal and that she must be a team member. Her demonstrated knowledge of benchmarking would be needed as a team resource.

The ball was now in Julie's court. Her team of supervisors had agreed to an approach, and her next actions were clear:

- Gain high-level support: She convinced her boss, Dr. Mike Schneider, Director of Transfusion Medicine, of the potential value of the benchmarking project. He agreed to become team **sponsor**.

- Request authorization: Julie explained to Dr. Schneider that his first task as team sponsor was to obtain the go-ahead from hospital top management. He agreed to write a memo to the hospital administrator outlining the problem, the study process, the cost, and the time commitments required of project team members.

- Recruit team: She worked with the hospital Quality Improvement Director and the directors of nursing, plant engineering, and finance to identify individuals who have demonstrated an interest in CQI and are trained in its methods. Names of volunteers were obtained for her to interview, and she selected three — one from each of the other departments — to work with Alberta and herself from the blood bank. The person chosen as the nursing

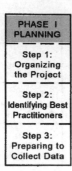

member was critical — she must represent **all** users of the blood bank's products.

- Legal: Julie promptly informed the hospital's legal counsel of the plan to contact other hospitals about operational performance. They agreed that he was to be made aware prior to major external interactions. His main caveat: there must be no mention of pricing when talking to other healthcare organizations.

**Figure 1. Benchmarking project proposal by Alberta Harrington.**

### Background

The Blood Bank is faced with many operational problems in a time of downsizing and efforts to reduce cost. All of the simple and obvious steps to improve operational efficiency have been taken. We need to find some new ways (to us) of doing our job that are already proven to work in other organizations. Benchmarking is "a tool for discovering and using the best approaches to getting work done." A number of possible subjects for a benchmarking project have been suggested. In the following, a specific subject is proposed and its choice explained.

### Proposed Subject

A Study of Blood Components Delivery Processes is proposed. It appears to be the best candidate for the following reasons:

1. Improvement in blood delivery will have an immediate positive impact on patient well-being.

2. It will lead immediately to elimination of blood component waste in the form of deliveries that exceed the 30-minute limit.

3. It will help eliminate hidden costs in the form of delayed patient therapies and tests that idle hospital personnel.

4. It will provide us with a solid factual basis (work process flow diagrams, process analysis) for the impending cost study being directed by Finance (see below).

5. If we select our benchmarking partners to include some who are doing liver and/or other transplants, we should be able to address our transplant blood demand/delivery problem automatically.

# The Blood Bank at Good Samaritan Hospital

## Other possible benchmarking subjects

1. Study of Cost of Blood Bank Operations—This is a very important task, but we are not ready to do it yet because we do not know our own costs in enough detail, and thus cannot do detailed comparisons with benchmarking partners. (Indeed, the proposed study of delivery processes will provide much of the framework for the development of our own cost profiles.) Also, it would probably be difficult to find benchmarking partners who are sufficiently clear about their own costs at this time.

2. Study of Leucocyte filtration—In some respects, this would be an ideal benchmarking topic because it is relatively limited in scope. It could even be done as a training exercise for more ambitious benchmarking projects, but its urgency and impact are not nearly as high as the delivery situation. Also, we have not yet settled down into a routine with our present process, and should gain more experience before we consider how to improve it.

**PHASE I PLANNING**

Step 1:
Organizing the Project

Step 2:
Identifying Best Practitioners

Step 3:
Preparing to Collect Data

## Project Description

1. Personnel—The project will require a team of five to six people representing the departments that are directly involved with blood components, with access to other professional specialists with knowledge of important technical details.

2. Time—The project should take three–four months, probably requiring about 1/2 day per week of team members' time.

3. Resources—It will be necessary to replace the time lost by the team members in benchmarking project activities, perhaps through overtime work by other staff members. Support from specialists can probably be absorbed into their regular work load if requests for their help are kept to a reasonable level.

4. Communications—To avoid misunderstanding and a negative response to the project, special pains should be taken to keep everyone with a stake in blood components delivery informed about the purpose and methodology of the benchmarking project. All stakeholders, especially Blood Bank people on the second and third shifts, should know that their knowledge and ideas will be needed and sought for many parts of the project.

5. Travel—It will probably be necessary to visit two or three other hospitals whose blood components delivery performance results are the best we have been able to find. The object of these visits will be to learn in much more detail how they are able to achieve such good results.

89

<table>
<tr><td>PHASE I<br>PLANNING</td></tr>
<tr><td>Step 1:<br>Organizing<br>the Project</td></tr>
<tr><td>Step 2:<br>Identifying Best<br>Practitioners</td></tr>
<tr><td>Step 3:<br>Preparing to<br>Collect Data</td></tr>
</table>

## MEETING WITH DR. YEAGER

Julie and Dr. Schneider decided that getting authorization for the project was a straightforward matter of explaining what they wanted to do, why, and how. Accordingly, they wrote a one-page letter to Dr. Charles Yeager, the hospital administrator, laying out their case. (See Figure 2)

---

**Figure 2. Letter of request.**

Date: March 1, 1995
To: Charles Yeager, M.D.
From: Michael Schneider, M.D.
      Julie Jones, Med. Tech.
Subject: Request for Project Authorization

1. The purpose of this letter is to request authorization to form a cross-functional team to study ways in which we can improve the processes by which blood components are distributed by the Blood Bank at Good Samaritan Hospital, and thus reduce errors and late delivery to the users. We believe that any improvements that we can make will lead to improved patient care and reduced cost of the Blood Bank's services in the hospital.

2. Because several different organizations are involved in distributing and using blood products, we propose that a project team be formed to do this, using the benchmarking process as the CQI tool. Benchmarking is designed to help a group with a work process problem to learn how other groups, who do the same work more effectively, are able to achieve better results. Using the benchmarking process will also help to ensure a receptive attitude toward better ways of doing things at Good Samaritan, so that the new knowledge can be put to work more quickly and easily.

3. We estimate that it will require a team of five people working roughly one half day per week (10% of their time) for three months to do the benchmarking project and bring the improved processes on line. We propose that the team include Elaine Robinson, R.N., Nursing Supervisor in the Burn Unit; William Smith Plant Engineering; James Hansen, Finance; Alberta Harrington from the Blood Bank; and Julie Jones as team leader. Dr. Schneider will serve as team sponsor and

---

advisor. Costs will be primarily in lost time on the job for team members, which we estimate to be no more than $10,000. This is to be compared with the estimated direct cost of mandated blood products discard (exceeding the 30-minute limit) in 1994 of over $50,000. Other costs driven by these delays (delayed or missed appointments in radiography, patient therapy, etc.) have not been estimated, but are believed to be even more wasteful.

A half-hour meeting has been scheduled in your office at 8:00 AM on March 3 to discuss this request in more detail and to answer any questions that you may have.

| PHASE I PLANNING |
| --- |
| Step 1: Organizing the Project |
| Step 2: Identifying Best Practitioners |
| Step 3: Preparing to Collect Data |

Dr. Yeager read their letter with interest and considerable skepticism. He had heard that benchmarking was another name for boondoggle travel, but he was keenly aware that Dr. Schneider and his blood bank supervisor were on a very important subject. Accordingly, he scheduled a full hour with them and probed the approach that they proposed fairly hard. He ended up complimenting them on how well they had thought through their intended approach, and gave the project a green light. As anticipated, he asked to be kept informed regularly by Dr. Schneider, particularly if it appeared that travel might be involved.

Dr. Schneider and Julie kept good notes of the meeting and the agreements reached. In their post-meeting discussion over coffee, they agreed that the things that had sold Dr. Yeager included their emphasis on the estimated dollar returns on the project's cost and the way they had handled possible travel needs. (See Figure 3)

## FIRST TEAM MEETING

The first meeting of the benchmarking team was intended to include discussions on:

- Project subject and scope.
- Team membership.
- Team activities.
- Schedule.

**PHASE I
PLANNING**

**Step 1:
Organizing
the Project**

**Step 2:
Identifying Best
Practitioners**

**Step 3:
Preparing to
Collect Data**

**Figure 3. Meeting with the director — agenda.**

(Annotated with notes from meeting; * indicates agreement)

- THE PROBLEM
  - Blood Bank overwhelmed by a combination of short staff, operational problems, need to accommodate new initiatives, and the imminent cost study.
  - Most worrisome is the problem of late deliveries and errors in blood products delivery. Hits patient care, operating costs, and staff morale.

- THE PROPOSED APPROACH
  - Explained what benchmarking is and why it is the indicated process.
  - Made argument for a team approach, and the importance of management support across organizational lines.
  - Gave a rough idea of the expected sequence of events.
  - Explained need for a team sponsor; Dr. Schneider's great willingness to serve.

- PROJECTED BENEFITS
  - Estimated annual savings of $50,000 from scrap reduction of blood products alone.
  - Crude estimate of cost of delays in radiography alone.
  - Referenced other delays: physician time lost, delayed therapies, start of surgery.
  - Cited data on delays for x-rays and other tests as the second most important cause of patient dissatisfaction at Good Samaritan. Touched lightly on highly competitive hospital business climate.

  * *AUTHORIZATION TO PROCEED GIVEN; DR. SCHNEIDER TO BE TEAM SPONSOR*

- RESOURCE REQUIREMENTS

  TIME
  - 1/2 day per week for three months for five people named. Estimated cost no more than $10,000.
  - Mentioned need for released time and authorization to cover with overtime and perhaps contract labor.
  - Mentioned desire to do much of the work outside meetings—use meetings for group-mandatory activity.
  * *OK FOR TEAM OF FIVE*
  * *CLOSE MONITORING REQUIRED FOR OTHER TIME EXPENDITURES*
  * *COVERING: OVERTIME ONLY, NOT TO EXCEED $8,000*

TRAINING
- Need one day equivalent of team training and team-building.
- Believe we can follow benchmarking process from published materials.
* *OK UP TO FOUR HOURS*

FACILITATOR
- Believe we will need some help occasionally from a consulting facilitator, but use self-facilitation as much as possible.
* *OK FOR CONSULTATION ONLY*

TRAVEL
- Described concept of Site Visit. Acknowledged that it was expensive, and not always necessary.
- Requested authorization in principle, with specific needs to be determined.
* *AUTHORIZATION ON HOLD FOR NOW*

- PROJECT SCHEDULE
  - Explained that a detailed work plan has not been produced yet, should be a team effort tied tightly to the objectives and scope of project.
  - Cited experience from the outside that a stable work plan is usually not achieved until second/third meeting of the team. (This discussion did not proceed smoothly.)
  * *TEAM CHARTER TO COMPRISE TEAM WORK PLAN AND COVER MEMO*
  * *PROGRESS TO BE REPORTED ONCE A MONTH INFORMALLY BY DR. SCHNEIDER*

- SUMMARY
  - J.J. hit hard on urgency of blood delivery issue, cost of scrap, and relatively small cost of requested resources. Dr. Y. seemed to take a personal interest in team approach and prospects for success.

| PHASE I PLANNING |
| --- |
| Step 1: Organizing the Project |
| Step 2: Identifying Best Practitioners |
| Step 3: Preparing to Collect Data |

However, not much got done at this first meeting. The initial meeting of any cross-functional group of this sort seldom do, because the group is not yet a real team:

- Group members probably don't know each other well enough.

- Group members don't share a similar knowledge of the facts, or attitude toward the relative significance of these facts.

- They probably don't agree on some aspects of team objectives.

**PHASE I**
**PLANNING**

**Step 1:**
**Organizing**
**the Project**

**Step 2:**
**Identifying Best**
**Practitioners**

**Step 3:**
**Preparing to**
**Collect Data**

- They may be looking for hidden agendas.
- Members are unsure of how much freedom they have.

The usual result of this atmosphere of uncertainty is inconclusive discussions and all-around frustration. That is what happened here. The group did not accept Julie's statement of what the team objectives should be, and were therefore unable to make progress on planning team activities. Julie Jones, Mike Schneider, and Alberta Harrington should not be blamed for this poor start. CQI is still in its early days at Good Samaritan, and none of these people had sufficient experience in the dynamics of cross-functional teams tackling very sensitive subjects to predict the course of the meeting. The main accomplishment of the meeting was to identify some action items, which Julie agreed to take on. (See Addendum for the Minutes of this and all other team meetings.)

## Julie's Actions: Team Building

First, Julie went to the hospital's trained facilitator. Their discussion touched on many of the principles of team building and teamwork, and together they came up with an agenda for a training/team building session that looked like this:

### Team-Building Meeting Agenda

- Around the table — personal statements
  - short biographical sketch
  - why I volunteered
  - what I know about the problem so far
- Short game designed to show the benefits of pooled knowledge
- Short tutorial on the practice of benchmarking, strong emphasis on Step 1: Organizing the Project
- Short game designed to show the benefits of a common goal
- Around the table — objectives and goals
  - Individual views on overall objective and team goal
- Consensus on project goal
- How the team should operate (Roles and Responsibilities). Tangible outputs expected:
  - meeting ground rules
  - meeting roles

Because the desired atmosphere was one in which people were encouraged to speak their piece without being rushed, this agenda was ambitious for the amount of time budgeted. However, the facilitator said he thought it would work.

| PHASE I PLANNING |
| --- |
| **Step 1: Organizing the Project** |
| Step 2: Identifying Best Practitioners |
| Step 3: Preparing to Collect Data |

## THE BENEFITS OF AN INVESTMENT IN TEAM-BUILDING

Experience has shown that an investment in team-building made at the beginning will usually pay big dividends in team effectiveness later.

People volunteer for team projects for a variety of motives ranging from desire for career exposure to a hot new fad to genuine concern with fixing the operational problems — as in the blood bank case. Somehow they must become a team with a common purpose and a willingness to trust each other and work together.

Having a common purpose is particularly important in a benchmarking project, because all team members must be able to support the project by advocating it in their home organizations. Also, everyone else who has a stake in the outcome of the project has to be made to feel that the project is focused on the work, not on a power struggle or some other side-show, and that their interests are adequately represented. These requirements can be met reliably only if the project objectives, the team work process, and the team composition are fully agreed within the team.

Experience has also shown that team-building sessions without an actual work focus are likely to be futile in a healthcare environment. People are just too busy, too practical, and too results-oriented. The agenda shown here deals with that need in four ways:

1. In a playlike atmosphere, people are reminded somewhat subtly that the problem they are about to work on is beyond the powers of any one of them,

| PHASE I |
| PLANNING |
| Step 1: |
| Organizing |
| the Project |
| Step 2: |
| Identifying Best |
| Practitioners |
| Step 3: |
| Preparing to |
| Collect Data |

but that the **team** stands a much better chance of coming up with a workable solution.

2. A necessary background tutorial is presented.

3. The group resolves differences about the overall objective and the project goal.

4. The group produces an output — the rules of its own self-governance.

### Julie's Actions: Supplementary Participation

Julie went to the Vice President of Nursing Services and the Director of Plant Engineering and explained the need to ensure the availability of additional informal representation from their organizations, plus the need for access to special expertise on occasion. When these stakeholders understood that satisfying the requests would enhance the quality of the team's conclusions and recommendations, each agreed to cooperate. They asked, however, that all requests be channeled through their respective offices for the sake of good order.

### Julie's Actions: Draft Work Plan

Knowing from experience that a project work plan and schedule are essential to success, Julie agreed to prepare a first cut at a **work plan** and schedule at the initial team meeting. She and Alberta drafted this plan, purposely leaving important details for team discussion at the next team meeting, since the other team members had shown that they wanted a hand in preparing the plan. Although she recognized that the plan would change as they went along, it was better to have a plan, however iffy, than to just wing it.

The team-building session took place two days before the scheduled second team meeting, and went smoothly. All those present had the basic CQI training, and understood the value of alignment to a single goal. They cooperated fully with the facilitator as he led them to consensus on the project's goal, and produced a creditable start on the team rules for self-governance.

## SECOND TEAM MEETING

After the reading of the Minutes of the first meeting (Addendum), the first item on the agenda was to revisit the rules for self-governance developed at the team training session. The group unanimously adopted the set of meeting process ground rules drafted at that session, including a "no-substitutes" rule that had been controversial at the time. A pledge to do as much work outside the meetings as possible to make best use of meeting time was also added. Julie felt particularly good about this pledge, because to her it demonstrated a commitment of the most practical kind (Figure 4).

The Meeting Roles draft was also quickly adopted (Figure 5).

With this bit of momentum, the team next tackled the item that had stalled progress at the first meeting: project objectives and scope. Both the nursing and the finance representatives had wanted to include liver transplant blood usage and white cell filtration. The group now revisited the consensus it developed at the team-building session and reached a somewhat more restricted majority decision (4:1) to include blood products usage in transplants, but not to include leucocyte filtration. Elaine Robinson, the nursing representative, was the hold-out advocate for the filtration process because of input she had received from her colleagues on one of the nursing units, but she agreed to support the majority vote, making it a consensus.

Everyone agreed, however, when Jim, the finance person, pointed out that the objective/scope discussion would have gone a lot faster if there had been a more detailed description of what management expected the project to deliver — a list of the items that should be in the project report. Alberta responded by saying that what he was asking for was a list of **Requirements for Success** for the project. Julie agreed to prepare a draft list for discussion at the next team meeting, adding that it might also come in handy when deciding what they wanted to find out from their benchmarking partners.

Per the agenda, they next took up the issue of team membership: how to balance the need for expert input against the need for

| PHASE I PLANNING |
| --- |
| Step 1: Organizing the Project |
| Step 2: Identifying Best Practitioners |
| Step 3: Preparing to Collect Data |

| PHASE I PLANNING |
| --- |
| Step 1: Organizing the Project |
| Step 2: Identifying Best Practitioners |
| Step 3: Preparing to Collect Data |

**Figure 4. Meeting ground rules.**

MEETINGS WEDNESDAY MORNING, 9:00 – 11:00 A.M.

(MEETING EVERY WEEK OR EVERY OTHER WEEK, DEPENDING UPON TIME REQUIRED TO COMPLETE HOMEWORK)

PUNCTUAL ATTENDANCE, COME TO THE MEETING PREPARED

STRIVE TO MINIMIZE INTERRUPTIONS DURING MEETING

APPROPRIATE NOTICE OF ABSENCE—VOTING PROXY TO ANOTHER TEAM MEMBER WHERE FEASIBLE

NO SUBSTITUTES

STICK TO THE AGENDA AND ITS TIME ALLOCATIONS

MINUTES DISTRIBUTED WITHIN TWO DAYS AFTER MEETING

MINUTES RECORD *ONLY* MAJOR DECISIONS, NEXT MEETING'S AGENDA, AND ACTION ASSIGNMENTS, EXCEPT UPON AGREEMENT AT MEETING

EACH MEMBER IS RESPONSIBLE FOR TEAM PROGRESS

PRE-READING DISTRIBUTED AT LEAST TWO DAYS AHEAD OF TIME

DISAGREEMENT OK, BUT CRITICIZE IDEAS, NOT PERSONS

TRY HARD FOR CONSENSUS, BUT SUPPORT THE MAJORITY DECISION EVEN IF YOU DISAGREE WITH SOME DETAILS

EVERYONE USE THE CQI MEETING FACILITATOR SKILLS

WORK STRATEGY:

DO AS MUCH WORK AS POSSIBLE OUTSIDE THE MEETINGS, RESERVING MEETING TIME FOR REFINING AND REACHING AGREEMENT ON ASSIGNED ACTIONS

**Figure 5. Meeting roles.**

PHASE I
PLANNING

Step 1:
Organizing
the Project

Step 2:
Identifying Best
Practitioners

Step 3:
Preparing to
Collect Data

- PROPOSED MEETING ROLES AND RESPONSIBILITIES:
  - DISCUSSION LEADER—Encourages active participation from each member, coordinates and covers the agenda, directs and monitors discussion, begins and ends on time.
  - SCRIBE—Creates a visual verbatim record of information during meetings on a flip-chart or white-board. Prepares minutes of the-meeting per Meeting Ground Rules (q.v.)
  - TIMEKEEPER—Assures that time constraints are clear, "sounds the alarm" if time is running short, helps discussion leader keep meeting on time for each agenda item.
  - PROCESS CHECKER—Ensures that discussion is proceeding smoothly, not hanging up on procedural points. When needed, suggests process tools to use. Leads meeting critique at end of meeting.

- PROPOSED ROLE ASSIGNMENTS
  - Rotation of the roles in sequence, from process checker to timekeeper to scribe to discussion leader and back to process checker.

- PROPOSED STARTING ROLES
  - DISCUSSION LEADER: ALBERTA
  - SCRIBE: JIM
  - TIMEKEEPER: BILL
  - PROCESS CHECKER: ELAINE
  - TEAM LEADER: JULIE (PERMANENT)

- ROLE SUBSTITUTES
  - No substitutes. If absence is unavoidable, individual is responsible to get another team member to cover

- OUTSIDE FACILITATOR
  - Try to get along without one. If help becomes indicated, Julie to arrange

- INVITED GUEST EXPERTS
  - Inviting host responsible for facilitating presentation and discussion. Also responsible to explain procedures to guest prior to project meeting.

**PHASE I
PLANNING**

**Step 1:
Organizing
the Project**

**Step 2:
Identifying Best
Practitioners**

**Step 3:
Preparing to
Collect Data**

small team size. Julie described the conversations with the Vice President for Nursing Services and the Director of the Plant Maintenance Department in which she had received assurances of their cooperation, mentioning that Dr. Schneider had supported her with telephone calls to both parties. Rules for "guest expert appearances" had already been adopted (see Figure 5) as a way of benefiting from meeting attendance by specialists in particular areas as needed, but without expanding the team to an unwieldy size, so no further action was required.

The Team Work Plan was on the agenda, but not covered due to time running out — the team was still learning how to work together efficiently. They did establish the *next* agenda, however, to include the Work Plan draft and the Requirements for Success draft, plus other items.

## THIRD TEAM MEETING

At its third meeting the team took up two major topics: the Requirements for Success strawman and the Team Work Plan draft.

Discussion of the list of Requirements for Success (Figure 6) drafted by Julie, was a huge success. Julie fleshed out with measurable detail the general statement of objective contained in the letter to Dr. Yeager seeking project authorization (Figure 2):

> *"... study ways in which we can improve the processes by which blood components are distributed by the Blood Bank at Good Samaritan Hospital, and thus reduce errors and late delivery to the users ... improvements ... will lead to improved patient care and reduced cost...."*

Using the draft as a departure point, the group added a number of details regarding the kinds of benchmarking partners they would be seeking (e.g., hospitals with a comparable numbers of beds). The discussion also brought recognition that benchmarking partners should have comparable facilities. Good Samaritan is housed in a 10-story building, computerized, but with no fiber-optic LAN. The list of success criteria was indeed proving to be a useful tool.

**Figure 6. Requirements for success.**

| |
|---|
| **PHASE I PLANNING** |
| **Step 1: Organizing the Project** |
| **Step 2: Identifying Best Practitioners** |
| **Step 3: Preparing to Collect Data** |

To be successful, the Blood Products Delivery Benchmarking Project must meet the following requirements:

1. Provide data on the *best delivery times* for all commonly used blood components that we can find in the U.S. among *institutions in similar circumstances.*

   a. Large size (500 + beds)

   b. Teaching hospital, preferably doing liver and/or heart-lung transplants

   c. Blood Bank delivers at least 40,000 units of transfusion products per year

   d. Computerized order processing

   e. Up-to-date pneumatic tube transport system

   f. Having a documented record of superior performance, preferably with a record of continuous improvement in a CQI environment

2. Provide data on the *range of delivery times* achievable by the best practitioners.

3. Provide data on the *total cost* of delivery among the best practitioners.

4. Provide data on the *cost of delays and replacements* for the best practitioners.

5. Provide detailed knowledge of the *work processes* by which these superior delivery times are achieved.

6. Provide detailed understanding of the *sources of delays and replacements* in delivery that have been discovered and eliminated by the best practitioners.

7. Provide workable recommendations for improving blood components delivery at Good Samaritan.

---

Coming to full agreement on the Requirements for Success solidified alignment of the team around the essential information the project was seeking. Everyone began to see that this list would become the guiding genius of the project.

The project work plan draft prepared by Julie and Alberta was scrutinized carefully for feasibility. The importance of doing most of the work outside team meetings became evident, and the team adopted the plan with the understanding that it might need revision at some point (Figure 7).

101

**Figure 7. Project plan.**

| PHASE I PLANNING |
| --- |
| **Step 1:** Organizing the Project |
| **Step 2:** Identifying Best Practitioners |
| **Step 3:** Preparing to Collect Data |

WEEK  3 — Develop criteria for selecting benchmarking partners
           Discuss contents of questionnaire

WEEK  4 — Prepare list of potential benchmarking partners
           Prepare first draft of questionnaire

WEEK  5 — Identify screener question
           Contact potential partners with screener

WEEK  6 — Pilot questionnaire internally

WEEK  7 — Finalize questionnaire

WEEK  8 — Mail questionnaire

WEEK  9 — Respond to inquiries from partners

WEEK 10 — Compile questionnaire results

WEEK 11 — Identify site visit issues
           Schedule site visits

WEEK 12 — Site visits

WEEK 13 — Draft recommendations

WEEK 14 — Sell recommendations internally

WEEK 15 — Finalize recommendations

WEEK 16 — Presentation to administrator and medical director

Having agreed to do the project work outside team meetings, the group gave itself the following **homework assignments** for the next meeting:

- All to search for possible benchmarking partners.

- All to develop lists of suggested questions for the questionnaire to be given to benchmarking partners. The team agreed to use the Requirements for Success list (Figure 6) as a guide to developing lists of possible questions.

- Julie and Dr. Schneider to sign off on the **team charter**, a memo based on the Work Plan and the Requirements for Success list.

The team was very busy after the third meeting. In the search for possible benchmarking partners, team members used contacts in

AABB, ASCP, and other professional societies to identify qualified and receptive hospitals. Dr. Schneider also provided several suggestions from his extensive list of contacts. As partner desirability criteria they used the "institutions in similar circumstances" description (size, number of transfused components, liver, and/or heart-lung transplant program) in Figure 6, plus a record of superior performance in blood components delivery, and, of course, an indication of desire to participate.

Team members also generated questions that they thought belonged on the questionnaire, again using the "Requirements for Success" list in Figure 6. Per agreement, these questions were sent to Alberta a few days before the next meeting for assembly.

After Ms. Jones and Dr. Schneider agreed on the content of the charter memo, it was issued with copies to all team members (Figure 8).

## FOURTH TEAM MEETING

This meeting had two agenda items — benchmarking partners and first draft questions for the questionnaire.

*Potential benchmarking partners.* Team members used their contacts to identify a total of 20 "live ones" and discussion using the partner desirability criteria in Figure 6 reduced this to a list of 10 clear front-runners for more serious consideration.

*First draft questions.* Alberta's consolidation work on individual lists proved very valuable. She had organized the individual submissions into possible topic areas and eliminated duplicate questions, which facilitated critical discussion of what they had so far.

Many of the questions focused on information the team was chartered to obtain:

- On which shift do you experience the greatest percentage of errors and delivery delays?
- What are the statistics of your actual delivery times *vs.* standard?
- What is the distribution of errors and delays by proximal cause?

PHASE I
PLANNING

Step 1:
Organizing
the Project

Step 2:
Identifying Best
Practitioners

Step 3:
Preparing to
Collect Data

| |
|---|
| **PHASE I PLANNING** |
| **Step 1:** Organizing the Project |
| **Step 2:** Identifying Best Practitioners |
| **Step 3:** Preparing to Collect Data |

**Figure 8. Team charter.**

Date: March 24, 1995
To: Michael Schneider, M.D.
From: Julie Jones, MT
Subject: Benchmarking Team Charter

The purpose of this memo is to document our agreement that a benchmarking team composed of Elaine Robinson, R.N.; William Smith, PE; James Hansen, CPA; Alberta Harrington, MT, and I will benchmark blood components delivery processes over an estimated four-month period, beginning on March 10. Limited consultation from expert colleagues has been authorized as well. You have agreed to be team sponsor. The team will spend approximately one half-day per week on the project, and incur out-of-pocket expenses not to exceed $8,000 (not including travel, which remains open). The Project Work Plan is outlined on Att. 1. It may be subject to modification.

The Blood Products Delivery Benchmarking Project will address the following requirements:

1. Provide data on the *best delivery times* for all commonly used blood components that we can find in the U.S. among *institutions in similar circumstances*, i.e.:

    a. Large size (500 + beds)

    b. Teaching hospital, preferably doing liver and/or heart-lung transplants

    c. Hospital transfuses at least 40,000 units of blood components per year

    d. Computerized order processing

    e. Up-to-date pneumatic tube transport system

We will be seeking partners having a documented record of superior performance, preferably with a record of continuous improvement in an institutional CQI environment.

2. Provide data on the *range of delivery times* achievable by these best practitioners.

3. Provide data on the *total cost* of delivery among the best practitioners.

4. Provide data on the *cost of delays and replacements* for the best practitioners.

5. Provide detailed knowledge of the *work processes* by which these superior delivery times are achieved.

6. Provide detailed understanding of the *sources of delays and replacements* in delivery that have been discovered and eliminated by the best practitioners.

7. Provide workable recommendations for improving blood components delivery at a cost not to exceed two years' savings.

Attachment—Project Work Plan (see Figure7—Ed.)

104

- How have these numbers trended over time?
- If the trend has shown improvement, what actions led to these improvements?
- May we have copies of the flow charts for your major work processes?

Many others addressed in rather more general terms how the work gets done:

- What training do new employees of the Blood Bank receive?
- What in-service training do they receive? How is it scheduled?
- What special provisions are made for training in new procedures?
- How frequently do you hold managerial staff meetings in the BB? All-hands staff meetings?
- What frequency of formal communications do you maintain with other support and supply operations?
  - Transportation
  - Business office
  - Blood supply (e.g., Red Cross)
  - Equipment supply/maintenance, re-agent supply

There were a few questions about the hospital's culture:

- Is your hospital using CQI?
  - If so, for how long?
  - Have all BB employees been trained in CQI?
- Do you measure employee satisfaction?
  - If so, how often?
- Do you measure user satisfaction?
  - If so, how often?
- What frequency of formal communications do you maintain with users?
  - OR's
  - Patient care units
  - ED

PHASE I
PLANNING

Step 1:
Organizing
the Project

Step 2:
Identifying Best
Practitioners

Step 3:
Preparing to
Collect Data

PHASE I
PLANNING

Step 1:
Organizing
the Project

Step 2:
Identifying Best
Practitioners

Step 3:
Preparing to
Collect Data

However, while there were a few redundant questions, some topics were not covered at all. There were some questions irrelevant to the project goal:

- How is the budget of the Blood Bank established?
- Is the Blood Bank required to show an internal "profit"?

and a need for deeper penetration in most areas. In short, it was a typical first attempt.

During the discussion, the team discovered and broke out from the main body of questions a set of **"screener questions,"** to be used in selecting a final list of benchmarking partners (Figure 9).

Realizing that quick action was required, the team organized the questions into various sections, one directed at the blood bank, others at specific user groups, etc., to make it easier for the benchmarking partners to answer the questionnaire. They also did some on-the-spot wordsmithing, but did not allow themselves to be sucked into hair-splitting debates about wording. Instead, Jim volunteered to finish pulling the draft questionnaire together.

**Figure 9. Screener questionnaire.**

- About how many units of blood components do you transfuse in a typical year?
- Do you obtain your blood products from the Red Cross or a community blood bank?
- Do your modes of delivery include:
  - pneumatic tube?
  - insulated blood cooler?
  - dumb-waiter?
  - messenger?
- Is your hospital housed in a one/two-story campus or a high-rise building?
- What is the total FTE employment in your blood bank?
- Do you do liver, heart-lung, or bone-marrow transplants?
- Do you keep track of delays and waste in delivery of blood products in the hospital?
- Do you track the functional area involved in instances of delay and waste?
- Do you make estimates of the cost of delays and waste in the work of the blood bank?

They were somewhat surprised at their productivity during the meeting and decided that they were ready to try out their main questionnaire draft in-house. Accordingly, it was agreed that there would be no meeting next week — instead, they would *pilot* the draft questionnaire.

Another action that they agreed should go on at the same time was that the persons who had made the original contacts with the 10 most promising potential partners would administer the screener questionnaire by telephone to identify serious mutual interest. Everyone agreed to follow the same protocol in administration of the screener questionnaire:

- Be sure you are talking to the right person. Your initial contact is probably someone you know, but not necessarily the person who can or should agree to a benchmarking partnership.

- Explain what we are trying to do in as much detail as the person you are calling wants. Then go over the screener questions.

- If the answers meet our criteria, say that you believe Good Samaritan can learn from the other party's experience. Say that your own hospital may have experience that might be useful to the other party as well, and that a partnership of shared experiences is what we are seeking.

- Explain what will be involved: a questionnaire that will take some effort to complete, possibly a request for a site visit, a fully confidential report profiling the operations of all participants — each one a leading blood bank — and an invitation for a reciprocal visit.

Things did not go quite as expected, however. The in-house questionnaire pilot was a real eye-opener and it slipped the schedule by a week.

## FIFTH TEAM MEETING

This meeting had three agenda items: Final selection of benchmarking partners, Results of the questionnaire pilot, and Finalization of the Questionnaire.

| PHASE I PLANNING |
| --- |
| Step 1: Organizing the Project |
| Step 2: Identifying Best Practitioners |
| Step 3: Preparing to Collect Data |

PHASE I
PLANNING

Step 1:
Organizing
the Project

Step 2:
Identifying Best
Practitioners

Step 3:
Preparing to
Collect Data

*Benchmarking partners.* All contacts were made and 6 of the 10 organizations contacted showed sufficient interest to be included in the final selection process. Everyone felt that the screener questionnaire and process had proven very valuable in communicating with potential partners.

Before the meeting, Julie developed a decision process with several criteria for selecting the top choices from among the benchmarking partner candidates. The team's preliminary inquiries prior to the screening calls had established that all potential benchmarking partners were big enough (beds, transfusions, blood bank employment), were teaching hospitals doing transplant programs, were comparably computerized, and had a pneumatic tube system. Thus, there was nothing to discriminate among the candidates on any of these grounds.

What she chose instead was a set of four criteria where there might be important differences among the contenders. These included type of buildings, whether the organization does waste- and cost-tracking, plus overall level of performance. These she listed down one side of a flip chart, with columns for the potential partners (identified here simply as A, B, etc.) ranged across the top of the chart.

Based on the screening interviews, the group felt that the *level of enthusiasm* for the project and *proximity* should be added to the list of criteria, with the latter being a practical consideration if a site visit turned out to be important. This was easily done by adding them to the list in the column headed "Criteria."

Julie had left blank a column on her flip chart headed "Weighting." She explained to the group that obviously not all criteria were equally important, but she had been hesitant to decide on her own what the weightings should be. After discussion and voting, the group settled on a weighting scheme that they agreed was close enough for their purpose, which was to pick the top four from the list of six candidates.

Finally, she explained how she had assigned numerical rating values to such things as "building type" and "cost-tracking." She thought it was most important to *distinguish* among the contenders, and for this, small whole numbers were satisfactory. For example, if the building type is a high-rise (like Good Samaritan) it rates a "2," but a campus setting is not necessarily useless, so it rates a "1." She mentioned that in a scheme of this sort, the *most desirable* rating should always use the *same number*, otherwise it would obscure the significance of the weighting scheme. With this guidance the team quickly assigned numbers for "enthusiasm" and "proximity."

The group then pooled and compared the information about the potential partners line by line on the flip chart, assigning rating numbers as they went. The scribe then added the results, which are shown on Table 1.

| PHASE I PLANNING |
| :---: |
| Step 1: Organizing the Project |
| Step 2: Identifying Best Practitioners |
| **Step 3: Preparing to Collect Data** |

Table 1. Partner selection decision process.

| Criteria | Weighting | Potential partners | | | | | |
|---|---|---|---|---|---|---|---|
| | | A | B | C | D | E | F |
| Enthusiasm | (x2) | 2 | 1 | 2 | 1 | 1 | 1 |
| Proximity | (x2) | 1 | 2 | 2 | 2 | 0 | 2 |
| Building type | (x1) | 2 | 1 | 2 | 2 | 2 | 2 |
| Waste tracked | (x3) | 2 | 2 | 2 | 2 | 2 | 0 |
| Cost tracked | (x3) | 2 | 2 | 2 | 2 | 0 | 0 |
| Performance | (x3) | 2 | 1 | 1 | 2 | 1 | 1 |
| TOTAL | | 26 | 22 | 25 | 26 | 13 | 11 |

Notes:

1. The numbers in the matrix are rating values as follows:

| Enthusiasm | – High = 2; Medium = 1; Low = 0 |
|---|---|
| Proximity | – <200 miles = 2; 200 – 1000 = 1; >1000 = 0 |
| Building type | – High-rise = 2; Campus = 1 |
| Cost, waste tracked | – Yes = 2; No = 0 |
| Performance | – Very superior = 2; Superior = 1; Good = 0 |

2. The numbers in parentheses are the weighting factors for the importance of the various criteria, where High = 3, Medium = 2, and Low = 1.

3. Totals for each potential partner are obtained by multiplying the numbers in its column in the matrix by the weighting factor in each row and adding the resulting weighted ratings.

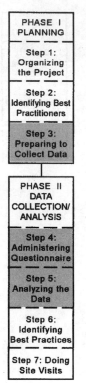

PHASE I
PLANNING

Step 1:
Organizing
the Project

Step 2:
Identifying Best
Practitioners

Step 3:
Preparing to
Collect Data

PHASE II
DATA
COLLECTION/
ANALYSIS

Step 4:
Administering
Questionnaire

Step 5:
Analyzing the
Data

Step 6:
Identifying
Best Practices

Step 7: Doing
Site Visits

There were three clear winners (A, C, and D), two clear losers (E and F), and one (B) that might have required further discussion if either E or F had been closer. As it was, the team selected the four frontrunners as benchmarking partners.

*Questionnaire pilot.* The in-house pilot had produced a bit of a shock: "We can't answer some of our own questions!" In order to get these answers, blood bank and user-group people had been required to flow-chart some work processes and to collect some critical data. This took considerable work, naturally, which is why meeting 5 was postponed. The good news was that Julie, Alberta, and Jim (the Finance member) all recognized that the work was basic to the forthcoming cost study and to quality improvement in general, and had to be done sometime anyway.

*Questionnaire.* One positive result from the in-house pilot was that thanks to good preparation there wasn't much wrong with the questionnaire itself that couldn't be quickly fixed. Perceiving this, Alberta and Jim had taken the initiative to make most of the fixes before the meeting. A few finishing touches were now added, and the questionnaire (Figure 10) was declared ready to be sent to the partners chosen by the ranking process described above.

It was agreed that Jim would send out the questionnaire by overnight mail (a subtle indicator of importance, they felt), and that the original contact person would follow up in two days with a phone call. It was also agreed that the next meeting would be in two weeks to give respondents ample time to work with the questionnaire.

## SIXTH TEAM MEETING

This meeting had a single agenda item — the questionnaire responses.

Three out of four of the responses were received on time; one was late, but promised for the next day. Alberta said that from her reading she gathered this was about par for the course.

# The Blood Bank at Good Samaritan Hospital

**Figure 10. Final questionnaire.**

I - TO BE ANSWERED BY BLOOD BANK CHIEF SUPERVISOR

1. What is the number of units of transfused blood products delivered by your Blood Bank per year, averaged over the past five years? _____

2. Do your modes of delivery include:
   – pneumatic tube? _____
   – insulated blood cooler?_____
   – dumb-waiter?_____. ___
   – messenger? _____

3. What percent of the time are Blood Bank personnel used for delivery when the pneumatic tube system is down? _____%

4. What is total FTE employment in your Blood Bank?

   _____

5. What is shift staffing by function? _____

   |                  | day | evening | night |
   |------------------|-----|---------|-------|
   | Supervisor       |     |         |       |
   | Bench test       |     |         |       |
   | Tech. specialist |     |         |       |

6. What is the academic background of your BB employees?

   High school _____%, AAS _____%, BS _____%, other _____%

7. How many weeks of training do new employees of the Blood Bank receive?

   _____

8. How much in-service training do they receive? How is it scheduled?

   _____
   _____

9. What special provisions are made for training in new and modified procedures? _____

   _____

10. How frequently do you hold supervisory staff meetings in the Blood Bank? _____ All-hands staff meetings?_____

11. Is your hospital using CQI?_____

   – If so, for how long? _____

   – Have all BB employees been trained in CQI? _____

12. Do you measure employee satisfaction? _____

   – If so, how often? _____

13. Do you measure user satisfaction? _____

   – If so, how often? _____

14. What frequency of formal communications do you maintain with users (and the principal mode of communication with each of these)?

|  | Frequency | Mode |
|---|---|---|
| – Surgical Services | | |
| – Medical Services | | |
| – ED | | |
| – OR's | | |

15. What frequency of formal communications do you maintain with other support and supply operations (and the principal mode of communication with each of these)?

|  | Frequency | Mode |
|---|---|---|
| – Engineering Dep't | | |
| – Computer services | | |
| – Blood supply (e.g., Red Cross) | | |
| – Biomedical Eng'g | | |
| – Re-agent supply | | |

16. What are your averages (minutes) for delivery time of blood products to users?

   – OR's _____

   – Surgical Services (incl. ICU) _____

   – Medical Services (incl. ICU) _____

– ED _____

– OPD's (adult and pediatric) _____

17. What are the limits (minutes) within which 95% of your actual deliveries take place?

    – OR's ____ to ____

    – Surgical Services (incl. ICU) ____ to ____

    – Medical Services (incl. ICU) ____ to ____

    – ED ____ to ____

    – OPD's (adult and pediatric) ____ to ____

18. What is the average total cost of one unit of each of the following products delivered to the user?

    | Packed RBC | _____ | – | Washed RBC | _____ |
    |---|---|---|---|---|
    | Platelets (conc) | _____ | – | Autologous | _____ |
    | Fr. fr. plasma | _____ | – | Whole blood | _____ |
    | Cryoprec | _____ | – | filt. RBC | _____ |

19. What is the average frequency per 100 orders for each of the following:

    – Time limit expired _____

    – Wrong product _____

    – Lost _____

    – Broken _____

20. Have these numbers shown an improvement trend over time?

    _____

21. If the trend has shown improvement, were there specific actions taken which led to these improvements?
    (Yes or No) _____

22. Do you do any of the following in-process Quality Assurance monitoring?

    – Late arrival reported _____

    – Broken package reported _____

    – Lost product reported _____

23. What is the total dollar cost of delivery delay for all blood components?  $_____

24. What percent of this cost is attributed to
    - Blood Bank materials & labor        _____%
    - OR downtime                         _____%
    - Ancillary services lost time        _____%
    - Other waste                         _____%

25. What is the total dollar cost of replacement orders for all blood components due to breakage? _____

**PHASE II
DATA
COLLECTION/
ANALYSIS**

**Step 4:
Administering
Questionnaire**

**Step 5:
Analyzing the
Data**

**Step 6:
Identifying
Best Practices**

**Step 7: Doing
Site Visits**

II – A SECTION CONSISTING OF 20 QUESTIONS TO BE FILLED OUT SEPARATELY BY NURSING SUPERVISORS IN OR's, MEDICAL AND SURGICAL SERVICES, ED, ICU's, AND UNIT SECRETARIES OF ADULT AND PEDIATRIC OPD's.

*Sample Question:* Do you adhere strictly to a 30-minute limit on elapsed time from blood components leaving refrigeration to transfusion into patient? _____

III – A SECTION CONSISTING OF 10 QUESTIONS TO BE FILLED OUT BY PLANT ENGINEERING'S PNEUMATIC TUBE SECTION.

Sample question: About how many times per month is there an interruption in the service of your pneumatic tube system? _____/mo.

IV – A SECTION CONSISTING OF 5 QUESTIONS TO BE FILLED OUT BY THE MESSENGER SERVICE.

Sample question: How much time elapses from receipt of a request for a messenger from the Blood Bank to messenger arrival at the Blood Bank dispensing window?_____ min.

---

Jim had made copies of the three returned questionnaires to hand out to everyone at the meeting, who pounced on them eagerly. In perusing the responses, team members discovered some impressive figures on short delivery times and small amounts of waste blood products due to delays. They also noted that the best performance was not confined to a single institution — for example, one hospital had best delivery times, another had lowest costs. One hospital (Mercy) had shown the most improvement in delivery time spread, but was still not the best. Although all of the group members loved to wallow around in data, in the interest of time they concluded this part of the discussion with the understanding that Jim and Bill would compile the results of all four responses and circulate them for study prior to the next meeting.

As can be imagined, there was considerable speculation on how some of this great performance was achieved. Accordingly, in preparation for the next meeting, the team members agreed to seek details by telephone from their benchmarking partners about the best practices revealed in the questionnaire responses. They realized, however, that such contacts might not tell them everything they needed to know about the work processes of the benchmark organizations. The team knew that they had no guarantee that site visits would be approved, but in case a strong need for face-to-face discussion of crucial practical details with the best practitioners emerged, they felt it was time to begin looking into the possibility. Julie volunteered to sound out the prospects for management support for site visit travel, using the raw input received so far. Team members would assess the desirability of site visits based on the outcomes of their telephone inquiries. They would also make inquiries about possible requests for consulting fees.

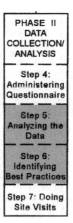

## SEVENTH TEAM MEETING

This meeting had two agenda items — analysis/discussion of the results and a site visit discussion.

*Compiled results.* Team members had already studied the compilation circulated before the meeting (Table 2), and quickly reached the conclusion that no one hospital was best at everything, Good Samaritan could learn something from all the partners. In fact, just knowing that other organizations had significantly better performance figures was valuable input all by itself.

Going into the details on Table 2, they noted that

- Mercy was a standout for service to OR's and for least cost of waste.

– Western Medical Center was best for service to OPD's and for least cost of breakage.

The team then compared Good Samaritan's performance vs. the benchmark:

– total cost of delivery delay was six times that of Mercy, the benchmark

– average turnaround time (TAT) was almost twice the benchmark. Also, the considerably narrower spreads (95% time) in delivery TAT for the other hospitals imply significantly different work and/or control processes

– spread in 95% times was over twice that of Mercy and Western Medical, the benchmarks

– cost of breakage was over 30 times that of Western Medical, the benchmark.

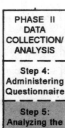

PHASE II
DATA
COLLECTION/
ANALYSIS

Step 4:
Administering
Questionnaire

Step 5:
Analyzing the
Data

Step 6:
Identifying
Best Practices

Step 7: Doing
Site Visits

Next the team stepped back a bit, ignoring for the moment interesting but probably minor points (e.g., they did not know what Western Medical meant when they talked about an "equivalent" TAT), and looked at the big picture. The work to date had confirmed that the blood components delivery problem at Good Samaritan comprised several problems:

– Order logjams at peak periods

– Delivery logjams at busy locations

– Breakage in the pneumatic tube system

– Constant firefighting by staff

– Poor user relations

Moreover, best practices discovered at one or more of the other hospitals had revealed solutions to each one, if they could be made to work at Good Samaritan:

– Routine orders placed in advance by OPDs

– Better tube system design and hardware

– User procedures reduce time-expired waste

– Better relations with all users

# The Blood Bank at Good Samaritan Hospital

**Table 2. Key results.**

|  | Mercy | University | West. Med | City Cent. | Good Sam. |
|---|---|---|---|---|---|
| Units transfused per yr, 5-yr ave. | 48K | 50K | 51K | 40K | 60K |
| Blood Bank FTE employees | 35 | 37 | 37 | 39 | 45 |
| **Turnaround time (TAT)[1], minutes** | | | | | |
| – average | 26 | 32 | 27 (eq.)[2] | 40 | 45 |
| – OR, 95% limits | 20-40 | 21-55 | 22-45 | 21-60 | 30-80 |
| – OPD, 95% limits | 22-55 | 21-55 | 21-40 | 21-60 | 30-80 |
| – ICU's, 95% limits | 21-45 | 21-55 | 21-40 | 22-55 | 30-75 |
| **Cost of Delay** | | | | | |
| – Total, $ | 350K | 800K | 450K | 900K | 2.0M |
| – BB, % | 75 | 50 | 70 | 45 | 50 |
| – OR, % | 23 | 45 | 29 | 53 | 45 |
| – floors, % | 2 | 5 | 1 | 2 | 5 |
| **Cost of breakage** | | | | | |
| – total, $ | 3K | 7K | <1K | 3K | 30K |
| **Replacement Frequency** | | | | | |
| – expired % | 4 | 6 | 5 | 6 | 14 |
| – broken % | .05 | 0.1 | .01 | .05 | 0.5 |
| – temp. lost % | .15 | 0.3 | 0.3 | .25 | ? |
| – wrong product % | .001 | .001 | .001 | .001 | .01 |
| – total % | 4.2 | 6.4 | 5.3 | 6.3 | >14.5 |
| **In-process monitoring** | | | | | |
| – late arrival | yes | yes | yes | yes | no |
| – lost, broken | yes | yes | yes | yes | no |

*Notes:*

[1.] Turnaround time (TAT) = Starting when order with sample arrives in Blood Bank and ending with beginning of transfusion into patient.

[2.] Eq. Not clear what Western Medical Center means by "Equivalent."

Perhaps most importantly, the team, rather than being discouraged by the state of affairs they had just documented, were fired with determination to fix the problems, because they saw the enormous overall benefits to be gained:

- Better patient satisfaction
- Much reduced waste
- Smaller blood bank staff
- Better blood bank staff satisfaction

PHASE II
DATA
COLLECTION/
ANALYSIS

Step 4:
Administering
Questionnaire

Step 5:
Analyzing the
Data

Step 6:
Identifying
Best Practices

Step 7: Doing
Site Visits

*Site visits.* Dr. Schneider kicked off this part of the discussion by announcing that he had just come from the CEO's office and that he had obtained the go-ahead for visits to two benchmarking partner sites. After the ensuing hubbub had died down, the team compared the benchmark numbers with the Project Success criteria (Figure 6) and talked about the results of their telephone discussions about best practices. They agreed on the need to visit Mercy Hospital (best delivery time for blood products to OR's, including liver transplant, and lowest overall cost due to waste), and Western Medical Center (best delivery service to OPD's, and smallest number of broken units).

The conversation then turned to the practical details of preparing for the visits, and homework actions were identified for the next meeting:

- Julie to schedule visits.
- Alberta to draft a site visit protocol based on her reading and discussions with the hospital's quality officer.
- All to identify site visit topics stemming from suspected deficiencies in Good Samaritan blood bank's work processes.

## EIGHTH TEAM MEETING

This meeting had two agenda items — site visit planning and (added agenda item) project report outline and assignments.

*Site visit planning.* The meeting got off to a good start, with Julie announcing that visits to Mercy and Western Medical Center had been set up consistent with the schedules of availability that team members had provided to her. Dr. Schneider was not certain of his availability (he was interested in going, but a backup had not yet been found for him).

The group then turned to discussion of the issues that they wished to address during the visits, focusing on obtaining a deeper understanding of the external work processes potentially most valuable to Good Samaritan.

The team members who would be responsible for covering each topic were chosen, based primarily on their ability to learn the most from what the visit team would be told.

*Site visit protocol.* Through reading, discussion with the quality officer, and her extensive experience observing accreditation site visits, Alberta was convinced that the most productive visits are the ones in which you are well prepared. When everyone is clear on what will be covered, who will do what, and when topics will appear on the agenda, things go better. Items that are easily handled with a phone call (like what *did* the folks at Western Medical Center mean by "equivalent turnaround time?"), should be clarified before the visit, keeping actual face-time for more complex and subtle discussion.

Accordingly, Alberta drafted a site visit process description and circulated it prior to the meeting. After some clarifying discussion and minor changes in wording, the site visit protocol was adopted. (See page 49, Step 7: Doing Site Visits.)

*Added agenda item: Report outline and assignments.* While reading Alberta's site visit process draft, Julie suddenly envisioned a way to speed up the project reporting process. Accordingly, with a small apology for being a bit disruptive, she passed out copies of a rough draft of a possible project report outline. She explained that she thought the site visits would be even more productive if people knew ahead of time how the issues were to be covered in the project report's recommendations for action, and who would have responsibility for preparing each recommendation. Julie then asked if the group felt ready to discuss this outline with an eye to volunteering for responsibility for the various sections of the report.

Everyone thought this was a good idea, and the assignments were quickly made and added to Julie's outline (Figure 11). It was

| PHASE II |
| DATA |
| COLLECTION/ |
| ANALYSIS |
| --- |
| Step 4: Administering Questionnaire |
| Step 5: Analyzing the Data |
| Step 6: Identifying Best Practices |
| Step 7: Doing Site Visits |

also agreed that everyone on the team had something to contribute to all aspects of the report, and that responsibility for writing included responsibility for folding in contributions from other team members. This point was made an addendum to Figure 11.

Julie received a bit of gentle kidding about having produced an outline that practically guaranteed the right "volunteers" for each report section, but all admitted that it was correct: it had the right structure for communicating with the various organizations in Good Samaritan who would be most affected by the benchmarking project's findings.

The meeting ended on a note of anticipation — no meeting next week: site visits instead.

## NINTH TEAM MEETING

The only item on the meeting agenda was the draft project report.

Informal communication among team members prior to the meeting had already established that the site visits had gone well. The good planning and preparation had paid off in solid information about how Mercy and Western Medical achieved such superior performance in delivery of blood products. Dr. Schneider had been able to make the trip to Western Medical Center, and was now in regular attendance at team meetings (a leading indicator of project success, one might say).

Team members, with admirable discipline, had all precirculated their section drafts to each other, with the exception of Section I, the Executive Summary, which Julie had not yet attempted to draft. The individual sections had proven easy to write — the simple structure of the outline allowed for the factual content to be presented in the style the author felt most comfortable with.

There was no wordsmithing at the meeting. Everyone had marked up (or promised to do so) each other's drafts with comments and suggestions on wording and returned them to the author for consideration for possible use.

This allowed the team plenty of time to focus on developing their recommendations. Since it was agreed at the beginning of the project that **everyone** must be committed to support **all** recom-

PHASE II
DATA
COLLECTION/
ANALYSIS

Step 4:
Administering
Questionnaire

Step 5:
Analyzing the
Data

Step 6:
Identifying
Best Practices

Step 7: Doing
Site Visits

PHASE III
INTEGRATION

Step 8:
Communicating
the Results

Step 9:
Establishing
Goals

mendations **fully**, it was important not to rush this discussion. They discussed the draft statements in each section in turn, referring continually to their Requirements for Success criteria (Figure 6).

Early in the meeting, Dr. Schneider urged the team not to strive for closure on the recommendations at this juncture. He pointed out that they would soon be seeking input from influential people who would have an immediate stake in what was about to be recommended. He warned the team against going to these opinion leaders with a *fait accompli*, creating a "take it or leave it" atmosphere that could work against obtaining the needed support.

**Figure 11. Project report outline.**

I   EXECUTIVE SUMMARY (Julie)
        = FINDINGS
        = RECOMMENDATIONS

II   RECOMMENDATIONS (All)

III   PROCEDURE (Julie)
        – TEAM MEMBERSHIP
        – BENCHMARKING PROCESS

IV   RESULTS
        – BLOOD BANK (Julie, Elaine)
        = FINDINGS
        = RECOMMENDATIONS
        – USERS (Elaine, Julie)
        = FINDINGS
        = RECOMMENDATIONS
        – PLANT ENGINEERING (Bill)
        = FINDINGS
        = RECOMMENDATIONS
        – MESSENGER SERVICE (Jim)
        = FINDINGS
        = RECOMMENDATIONS

APPENDIX (Alberta, Jim)
– QUESTIONNAIRE
– SITE VISIT PROTOCOL
– SCHEDULE
– TABULATED RESULTS (FOR FEEDBACK REPORTS TO
   BENCHMARKING PARTNERS)

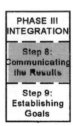

PHASE III
INTEGRATION

Step 8:
Communicating
the Results

Step 9:
Establishing
Goals

*Note:* Assignments are for draft preparation. All team members will have opportunity to contribute ideas and language to final version.

## WHAT MAKES FOR A SUCCESSFUL OPINION-LEADER INTERVIEW

The purpose of the interview meetings is to gain support from influential people for some recommended actions that *you* know about and that *they* do not — at least in any detail. You are most likely to get this support if you go in with the right *mind-set* and *preparation*.

- Give the key information about the project up front, for example, by providing a draft of the project report summary prior to the interview. (Be sure it is marked "draft.")

- Begin the interview by going over this information. Be completely factual.

- Be prepared for questions about all aspects of the project methodology, but don't volunteer nonessential detail.

- Be open to suggestions for improvement of the recommended action proposal. Listen carefully to comments of this sort, even when framed as criticisms of the proposal as it stands.

- Do not be defensive about the project. (This is hard — it's your baby and it is sometimes difficult to be objective.)

- The project was designed to have a specific scope. Don't make claims and promises not supported by your findings.

- Be prepared for viewpoints arising from professional and organizational biases.

- Flexibility may be required. Know what you can give up and what is crucial to success.

- Don't oversell.

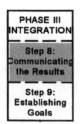

PHASE III
INTEGRATION

Step 8:
Communicating
the Results

Step 9:
Establishing
Goals

Dr. Schneider said that he would certainly do his part in explaining the results of the project to his peers on the executive committee. He stressed, however, that nothing would be as convincing as the individual team members meeting and objectively sharing their findings and conclusions with this group individually, particularly with those managers and directors who would be responsible for development and execution of the actual detailed action plans.

**Figure 12. Report executive summary.**

This benchmarking study compared the blood products delivery system at Good Samaritan Hospital to those of four similar hospitals (size, case mix, teaching, transplant programs). Key findings are displayed on Table A.

**Principal conclusions:**

1. Transfusion delay problems are costing Good Samaritan an estimated total of over $2M per year, compared to $350K for Mercy Hospital, which had the lowest cost in our study. The actual direct cost of replacement products charged to the Blood Bank budget at Good Samaritan is $1M, or approximately 50% of the total.

2. The balance of the cost of delay is indirect—OR delays account for 45%, and lost time for nursing staff accounts for 5%.

3. The Good Samaritan transfusion medicine system is not set up to cope with its huge variation (20 to >300 units/day) in orders for transfused products, while the other hospitals in our study are much better prepared to do so.

4. Our pneumatic tube system functions reliably with a moderate traffic level, but at higher volumes, performance on certain routes and stations deteriorates significantly below that of all four comparison hospitals.

5. Good Samaritan's breakage frequency is 50 times higher than that of Western Medical, which had the best breakage record of our benchmarking partners.

6. Our benchmarking partners all reported communications and cooperation with user groups superior to Good Samaritan's.

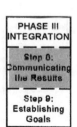

**Recommendations:**

Changes in the following areas are recommended, together with estimated costs of implementation.

   – Blood Bank (Procedural changes)—Cost: $0
   – Users (Procedural changes in OR's, Medical and Surgical Services, OPD's and ED) - Cost: $0
   – Pneumatic tube system (procedural changes and equipment modifications)—Cost: $100K capital, details on Table B.

See appropriate sections of report for detailed descriptions. (Detailed sections not included. - Ed.)

All of these recommended changes have been agreed to and are endorsed by the chiefs of the affected services, by the VP Nursing Services, by the Medical Director, and by the QA/I Department.

**Table A**

(Same as Table 2, p. 117 – Ed.)

**Table B**

Capital investment Proposal—Pneumatic Tube System

1. Addition of tube stations
   - surgical suites (3)          $60.0 K
   - ICU (1)                      $20.0 K

2. Modification of carriers
   - Modify all carriers        $ 4.0 K

3. Replace worn parts of system    $16.0 K
   TOTAL                         $100.0 K

*Notes:*
   a. Item 1 addresses delays due to heavy traffic.
   b. Item 2 addresses excessive breakage.
   c. Item 3 is essential maintenance work deferred in 1994.

---

**PHASE III
INTEGRATION**

Step 8:
Communicating
the Results

Step 9:
Establishing
Goals

---

Toward the end of the meeting, Dr. Schneider helped the group develop a list of key people for one-on-one discussions, and promised to help set these meetings up.

It was agreed there would be no meeting next week; individual appointments with key people would be the focus.

At the individual meetings with opinion leaders among the key stakeholders, everyone followed Dr. Schneider's advice:

- Be completely factual.
- Be open to other points of view, not defensive about team position as the only truth. Inevitably, some stakeholders will have differing views.
- Recognize individual sensitivities and built-in positions.

The result was that the project process and factual findings were accepted as credible, and the action recommendations were generally supported. Dr. Schneider informed his peers about the project's major findings and conclusions, which they received favorably. There was one partial holdout among the medical staff, who was willing, however, to support a fair trial before coming to a final position.

## TENTH TEAM MEETING

This meeting had three agenda items — results of discussions with opinion leaders, finalize report and recommendations, and communication with administrator.

*Opinion-leader discussions.* Team members compared notes and found that they had had very similar experiences. There was general agreement that following their sponsor's advice about behavior in discussion with the opinion leaders had been instrumental in their success.

*Finalize report/recommendations.* The team suddenly found that they were able to reconcile their previous differences regarding the recommendations. It seems that the need to explain the project and its results to people who were hearing the story for the first time, and from considerably different points of view, had helped to enlarge their own perspective. If the desire to improve operations is kept paramount, small differences fade in import. With very little ado, the executive summary of the report was approved, including the recommendations for changes in operations, and the proposed capital expenditures (Figure 12).

*Communication with Director.* Naturally, the team would have liked a meeting with the CEO, but recognized that he was a very busy man and chose to offer the report for his review and endorsement.

## EPILOGUE

There was no benchmarking team meeting with Dr. Yeager, the Good Samaritan Hospital CEO. Because of the excellent description of the work process, the findings and the rationale for the recommendations, and because all of the people and departments affected

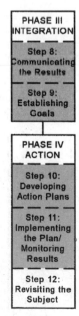

had already endorsed the recommended action plan, Dr. Yeager endorsed the proposed action plan without a meeting. Instead, he sent a brief memo to all the affected departments, urging their cooperation in implementing the proposed changes. However, to Julie Jones' intense gratification, he joined Dr. Schneider in hosting a wine-and-cheese party for the benchmarking team.

To date, the following actions are completed or underway:

1. Blood Bank personnel were all given copies of the benchmarking team report and attended meetings with Julie and Alberta at which any questions they had were fully addressed. The whole Blood Bank staff has attended workshops where they helped to prepare plans for improving Blood Bank relations with its customers, the users. A very recent user satisfaction survey yielded encouraging results in all areas except the ED. In response to the continuing issues with this group, a team of volunteers from both organizations has been set up to study Blood Bank service shortfalls to the ED.

2. Regularly scheduled transfusions to patients in the adult OPD are now called in to the Blood Bank far enough in advance so that the fulfillment of the orders takes place in a very orderly way. Replacement orders to the adult OPD are down 30% and the spread in the 95% time is down 50%.

3. Planning is taking place for the modifications in the tube system, and the 1996 capital budget will have a line item for these changes. As an interim measure, the OR's have adopted a version of the new order process in the adult OPD for some kinds of surgical patients, and the rush-hour backups in the Blood Bank are noticeably improved. Average downtime in the OR's has been reduced by 15%.

4. Led by Elaine Robinson, all nursing staff have taken an in-service course to acquaint them with the new procedure in which orders for blood components are not placed until transfusion lines have been placed in the patient.

| PHASE IV ACTION |
| --- |
| Step 10: Developing Action Plans |
| Step 11: Implementing the Plan/ Monitoring Results |
| Step 12: Revisiting the Subject |

Replacements are down by 30% in Medical Services and 20% in Surgical Services. Total savings in direct and indirect costs are estimated at over $20,000/mo.

5. The much-dreaded cost study turned out to be an easy exercise for the Blood Bank. The work processes were already flow-charted, and most of the cost elements had already been developed for the benchmarking project.

6. A reciprocal visit from representatives of Mercy and University Hospitals took place last week to trade process information about leucocyte filtration in the Blood Bank and to discuss mutual interests in best approaches to supplying transplant programs.

| PHASE I PLANNING |
| --- |
| Step 1: Organizing the Project |
| Step 2: Identifying Best Practitioners |
| Step 3: Preparing to Collect Data |

# ADDENDUM

## MINUTES OF FIRST MEETING

Date: March 8, 1995
Present: Alberta Harrington (Supervisor, Blood Bank); Bill Smith (Supervisor, Plant Maintenance); Elaine Robinson, R.N. (Nurse Supervisor, Burn Unit); Jim Hansen (Manager, Finance); Julie Jones, MPH (Chief Supervisor, Blood Bank, Chair)

### AGENDA

- Benchmarking subject/scope of project
- Team membership
- Team activities
- Schedule
- Next agenda

1. Meeting came to order at 2:15 P.M., Julie Jones as chairperson.

2. Project subject: Long discussion of benchmarking subject revealed lack of agreement about project scope and team objectives. General feeling that we did not use meeting time productively. Conclusion: we need to use the CQI processes more effectively.

ACTION: Julie to schedule a team-building session with facilitator staff.

PHASE I
PLANNING

Step 1:
Organizing
the Project

Step 2:
Identifying Best
Practitioners

Step 3:
Preparing to
Collect Data

3. Team membership: Agreed that we may need more representation from nursing staff (medical and surgical services, ICU and ED). Also need access to plant maintenance records, and advice about their use.

ACTION: Julie to contact VP, Nursing Services and manager, Plant Engineering, to discuss ways of ensuring good team communication with all stakeholder populations.

4. Team Activities: Discussion inconclusive. Not clear what we should be doing if we don't know we have full agreement about the scope of our subject. Agreement that we need a draft plan to focus discussion, however.

ACTION: Alberta and Julie to prepare a work plan draft.

5. Schedule: Same comment as for item #4.

## MINUTES OF SECOND MEETING

Date: March 17, 1995
Present: Alberta, Bill, Julie, Elaine, Jim

### AGENDA

1. Minutes of last meeting

2. Meeting process – rules and roles

3. Benchmarking subject/scope of project

4. Team membership

5. Draft team work plan

6. Next agenda

Meeting came to order at 9:00 A.M., Julie as chairperson

1. Minutes approved as submitted.

2. Meeting procedure — Discussion of suggestions from Quality Office facilitator staff provided at team training session, particularly "no substitutes" rule. Unanimous agreement to adopt the ground rules and meeting roles suggestions as presented.

3. Project subject/scope — Wide-ranging discussion of real purpose of the benchmarking project and how we will know it has been successful. Majority decision (4/1): scope to include blood products usage in liver (or heart-lung) transplant procedure, but not leucocyte filtration process.

128

ACTION, Julie: Prepare a strawman list of Requirements for Success for this project.

4. Team membership — Assurance of cooperation from Nursing and Maintenance Engineering. Unanimous agreement: Elaine (Nursing), Jim (Finance), and Bill (engineering) to obtain specialist consultations and "guest appearances" as needed by core team.

5. Team work plan — Not addressed; time constraint.

6. Next agenda

    1. Minutes of last meeting

    2. Requirements for Success Strawman

    3. Draft Team Work Plan

    4. Benchmarking partners

    5. Questionnaire Process

    6. Next agenda

Meeting ended at 11:40 A.M.
Respectfully submitted,
Alberta Harrington

| PHASE I PLANNING |
| --- |
| Step 1: Organizing the Project |
| Step 2: Identifying Best Practitioners |
| Step 3: Preparing to Collect Data |

## MINUTES OF THIRD MEETING

Date: March 24, 1995
Present: Alberta, Bill, Elaine, Jim, Julie

### AGENDA

    1. Minutes of last meeting

    2. Requirements for Success Strawman

    3. Draft Team Work Plan

    4. Benchmarking partners

    5. Questionnaire Process

    6. Next agenda

Meeting came to order at 9:00 A.M., Julie as chairperson

1. Minutes approved as submitted.

2. Requirements — Discussion of Julie's draft led to adding measures to Item #1, see below. Resulting list (copy attached) adopted as a guide to future work.

PHASE I
PLANNING

Step 1:
Organizing
the Project

Step 2:
Identifying Best
Practitioners

Step 3:
Preparing to
Collect Data

3. Work Plan — Clarifying discussion, especially about doability, led to unanimous commitment to finish outside assignments on schedule.

ACTION: JULIE to issue Team Charter memo to include Project Plan and Requirements for Success.

4. Partners — Discussion, using Requirements for Success list, especially the amplified version of item #1, to guide search for benchmarking partners.

ACTION: EVERYONE to provide list of possible candidates to Alberta for consolidation.

5. Questionnaire Process — Again, discussion focused on questions that will lead directly to a successful project.

ACTION: EVERYONE to bring to next meeting lists of questions for possible inclusion in questionnaire for benchmarking partners.

6. Next agenda

1. Minutes of last meeting

2. Benchmarking partners (cont.)

3. Questionnaire (first draft)

4. Next agenda

Meeting ended at 11:00 A.M.
Respectfully submitted,
Alberta Harrington

## MINUTES OF FOURTH MEETING

Date: March 31, 1995
Present: Alberta, Bill, Julie, Elaine, Jim

### AGENDA

1. Minutes of last meeting

2. Benchmarking partners (cont.)

3. Questionnaire (first draft)

4. Next agenda

Meeting came to order at 9:00 A.M., Julie as chairperson

1. Minutes approved as submitted.

2. Discussion of consolidated list of 20 potential benchmarking partners against desirability criteria (record of measured improvement in blood products delivery, liver transplant, size, teaching hospital). Decision to contact top 10 (willing, meet all criteria).

> ACTION: ALL to contact organizations you suggested, using screener questions discussed below.

3. Discussion of consolidated list of submitted questions (attached). Screener questions (attached) identified using desirability criteria.

> ACTION: ALL review and add to main questionnaire.
>
> ACTION: JIM to consolidate input and organize questionnaire ASAP for ease of response by partners.
>
> ACTION: BILL, ELAINE, AND JULIE to pilot questionnaire informally to see if we can answer our own questions.

4. Next agenda NOTE: NO MEETING NEXT WEEK!

   1. Minutes of last meeting
   2. Results of informal pilot
   3. Benchmarking partners (final)
   4. Questionnaire (final)
   5. Next agenda

Meeting ended at 11:00 A.M.
Respectfully submitted,
Alberta Harrington

| PHASE I PLANNING |
| --- |
| Step 1: Organizing the Project |
| Step 2: Identifying Best Practitioners |
| Step 3: Preparing to Collect Data |

## MINUTES OF FIFTH MEETING

Date: April 21, 1995
Present: Alberta, Bill, Julie, Elaine, Jim

### AGENDA

1. Minutes of last meeting
2. Results of informal pilot
3. Benchmarking partners (final)
4. Questionnaire (final)
5. Next agenda

| PHASE I<br>PLANNING |
| :---: |
| Step 1:<br>Organizing<br>the Project |
| Step 2:<br>Identifying Best<br>Practitioners |
| Step 3:<br>Preparing to<br>Collect Data |

| PHASE II<br>DATA<br>COLLECTION/<br>ANALYSIS |
| :---: |
| Step 4:<br>Administering<br>Questionnaire |
| Step 5:<br>Analyzing the<br>Data |
| Step 6:<br>Identifying<br>Best Practices |
| Step 7: Doing<br>Site Visits |

Meeting came to order at 9:00 A.M., Julie as chairperson

1. Minutes approved as submitted.

2. In-house piloting revealed gaps in knowledge of all groups' work processes. Intense effort has closed almost all of these gaps. General agreement on high future value of this activity.

3. Discussion of results of calls to potential benchmarking partners. Evaluated six positive responses against original desirability criteria (record of measured improvement in blood products delivery, liver transplant, size, teaching hospital) plus convenience of location and measure of enthusiasm. Decision to partner with top four. See attached decision scoring matrix results.

4. Discussion and wordsmithing of final questionnaire (copy attached). Decision to go with it. **THANKS** to Jim and Alberta for a great job of pulling questionnaire together.

   ACTION: JIM to mail out (FedEx) questionnaires with cover letters by contact person.

   ACTION: CONTACT PERSON to follow up in two days to reiterate offer of support in responding.

5. Next agenda **NO MEETING NEXT WEEK!**

   1. Minutes of last meeting
   2. Review questionnaire responses
   3. Next agenda

Meeting ended at 11:10 A.M.
Respectfully submitted,
Alberta Harrington

## MINUTES OF SIXTH MEETING

Date: May 5, 1995
Present: Alberta, Bill, Julie, Elaine, Jim

### AGENDA

1. Minutes of last meeting
2. Review questionnaire responses
3. Next agenda

Meeting came to order at 9:00 A.M., Julie as chairperson

1. Minutes approved as submitted.

2. Discussion of three responses (one not yet received, but promised within next two days). Very encouraging input.

   ACTION: JIM AND BILL TO compile results for analysis and further discussion.

   ACTION: ALL begin thinking about site visits (topics to be covered, possible requests for consulting fees, desire/availability for travel).

   ACTION: JULIE to discuss with Dr. Schneider the prospects for obtaining travel support from upper management.

3. Next agenda

   1. Minutes of last meeting

   2. Analysis/discussion of compiled results

   3. Site visits

   4. Next agenda

Meeting ended at 11:00 A.M.
Respectfully submitted,
Alberta Harrington

| PHASE II DATA COLLECTION/ ANALYSIS |
| --- |
| Step 4: Administering Questionnaire |
| Step 5: Analyzing the Data |
| Step 6: Identifying Best Practices |
| Step 7: Doing Site Visits |

## MINUTES OF SEVENTH MEETING

Date: May 12, 1995
Present: Alberta, Bill, Elaine, Jim, Julie, M. Schneider, M.D.

### AGENDA

1. Minutes of last meeting

2. Analysis/discussion of compiled results

3. Site visits

4. Next agenda

Meeting came to order at 9:00 A.M., Julie as chairperson.

1. Minutes approved as submitted.

2. Compiled results — Discussion of compiled results identified the key measures (attached) where one or more other institutions were significantly better in their blood products deliv-

ery performance than Good Samaritan. General agreement that we need to better understand the key work processes at Mercy Hospital and Western Medical Center.

(THANKS to Bill and Jim for compiling and distributing results in time for study prior to the meeting.)

3. Site visits – Dr. Schneider informed team that site visits to two organizations were authorized for up to three people each. Dr. Schneider has also been asked when the team's report will be ready.

ACTION: JULIE to schedule visits to Mercy and Western Medical.

ACTION: ALBERTA to draft a site visit process (protocol).

ACTION: ALL to identify issues for site visit and provide schedule of availability to Julie ASAP.

4. Next agenda

   1. Minutes of last meeting

   2. Site visit planning

   3. Next agenda

Meeting ended at 11:05 A.M.
Respectfully submitted,
Alberta Harrington

| |
| --- |
| **PHASE II** |
| **DATA** |
| **COLLECTION/** |
| **ANALYSIS** |
| **Step 4:** |
| **Administering** |
| **Questionnaire** |
| **Step 5:** |
| **Analyzing the** |
| **Data** |
| **Step 6:** |
| **Identifying** |
| **Best Practices** |
| **Step 7: Doing** |
| **Site Visits** |

## MINUTES OF EIGHTH MEETING

Date: May 19, 1995
Present: Alberta, Bill, Julie, Elaine, Jim, M. Schneider, M.D.

### AGENDA

   1. Minutes of last meeting

   2. Site visit planning

   3. Project report outline (added agenda item)

   4. Next agenda

Meeting came to order at 9:00 A.M., Julie as chairperson

   1. Minutes approved as submitted.

   2. Site visit planning — Julie announced that a site visit had been set up at Mercy Hospital for Julie, Alberta, and Bill on

May 23 and a visit to Western Medical for Elaine, Jim and perhaps Dr. Schneider on May 25. (If Dr. Schneider cannot go, Mary Q. Contrary, nursing supervisor in the OB/GYN surgical suite, has expressed willingness to go.)

Discussion of visit content produced lists of topics to be covered and responsible team members. Agreement also reached on responsibility for drafting individual sections of the benchmarking project report.

ACTION: ALL — Study your assigned topics and think about your report sections. (See attached assignment list.)

Discussion of the visit process produced the site visit protocol (attached) that will guide both site visits.

(THANKS to Alberta for a great job on the draft.)

3. Report outline — Julie handed out a strawman project report outline (apologies for no precirculation), and pointed out it might be useful as a thought-organizer for site visitors. Discussion produced minor modifications and agreement to follow the outline (attached) in preparing drafts of the report sections.

4. Next agenda NO MEETING NEXT WEEK — SITE VISITS AND REPORT DRAFTS

    1. Minutes of last meeting

    2. Draft benchmarking project report

    3. Next agenda

Meeting ended at 11:00 A.M.
Respectfully submitted,
Alberta Harrington

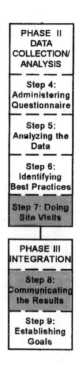

## MINUTES OF NINTH MEETING

Date: June 2, 1995
Present: Alberta, Bill, Julie, Elaine, Jim, M. Schneider, M.D.

### AGENDA

    1. Minutes of last meeting
    2. Draft benchmarking project report
    3. Next agenda

Meeting came to order at 9:00 A.M., Julie as chairperson

1. Minutes approved as submitted.

2. Draft project report — Discussion of circulated drafts led to consensus on key findings for executive summary, but some disagreement on recommended actions (see attached).

   Dr. Schneider led discussion of importance of building support for project's recommended actions from high-level stakeholders.

   – Agreement on need to obtain these opinion leaders' reactions to recommendations "before the concrete has set."

   – Also agreed that discussion of disagreements on recommendations should be deferred until after interviews with key stakeholders.

   ACTION: ALL make appointments with individuals suggested by Dr. Schneider to describe the benchmarking project's approach and results. Describe the recommended actions, explaining that they are still in draft, and ask for reactions.

3. Next agenda **NO MEETING NEXT WEEK — INDIVIDUAL APPOINTMENTS**

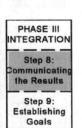

   1. Minutes of last meeting

   2. Results of discussions with opinion leaders

   3. Finalize report and recommendations

   4. Communication with Administrator

Meeting ended at 11:00 A.M.
Respectfully submitted,
Alberta Harrington

## MINUTES OF TENTH MEETING

Date: June 16, 1995
Present: Alberta, Bill, Julie, Elaine, Jim, M. Schneider, M.D. (part time)

### AGENDA

1. Minutes of last meeting

2. Results of discussions with opinion leaders

3. Finalize report and recommendations

4. Communication with Administrator

5. Next agenda

Meeting came to order at 9:00 A.M., Julie as chairperson

1. Minutes approved as submitted.

2. Discussions — Around-the-table established that the project's approach was already known (THANKS to Dr. Schneider!), the results are accepted, and most recommendations are well supported. Dr. Olsen, chief of surgery, suggested a different way of ensuring the avoidance of switched units at times of peak traffic into the OB/GYN surgical suite, but said he was willing to support giving the proposed approach a fair trial.

3. Report/recommendations — Project report and recommendations unanimously agreed by team (see attached).

4. Discussion of communication with Dr. Yeager.

ACTION: JULIE to canvass Dr. Y's wishes and arrange for communication of the team results and recommendations.

5. Next agenda

1. Minutes of last meeting

2. Communication with Dr. Yeager

3. Next agenda

Meeting ended at 11:00 A.M.
Respectfully submitted,
Alberta Harrington

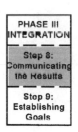

PHASE III
INTEGRATION

Step 8:
Communicating
the Results

Step 9:
Establishing
Goals

# Chapter 6

# Mercy Hospital Stroke Therapy Initiative

## Sponsor Perspective

*The sponsor of a benchmarking project is the person in a management position for whom the project is done. This person is the project's prime customer, and often its mentor.*

This case study is about a benchmarking project that is part of a program to introduce a major new emergency protocol. The new protocol involves the interactive participation of many different groups of providers and support personnel. The benchmarking project objective is to find the best possible process for getting all of these groups to change over to the new approach quickly and effectively.

Things to watch for in this case study are:

How the sponsor handles a benchmarking project that is one part of a multipart program.

How the sponsor can help to find and recruit benchmarking partners from outside healthcare.

| PHASE I PLANNING |
| --- |
| Step 1: Organizing the Project |
| Step 2: Identifying Best Practitioners |
| Step 3: Preparing to Collect Data |

How a schedule slip can happen and what to do about it.

How to inform and involve peers in executive-level management.

How to develop and use the team charter as a management tool.

How the sponsor can help recruit very busy people.

How to handle difficult questions in executive committee meetings.

Sponsor actions when the benchmarking team strays from its charter.

A good way to hand off benchmarking findings to the people who will have to carry out the recommended actions.

## THE SITUATION

Mercy Hospital is large tertiary-care teaching hospital serving a population scattered over a 50-mile radius. Several months ago Dr. Charles Smith, one of the leaders on the medical staff, approached John Jones, the CEO, about the possibility of Mercy being the innovator in its area in the clinical use of tissue plasminogen activator (tPA), a new and promising therapy for emergency treatment of ischemic stroke.

The idea for doing this came naturally to Dr. Smith — he is Clinical Professor of Neurology at the medical school with which the hospital is affiliated, and also Chief of Emergency Services at Mercy Hospital, an unusual combination of professional interests. Dr. Smith knew that Mercy felt it had a responsibility in the community to lead in the use of new therapies. This obligation was particularly strong for illnesses like stroke, with its widespread impact on the whole community's population.

When Dr. Smith raised the issue, Mr. Jones was quick to agree in principle, pointing out that the reputation of Mercy Hospital depended in part on such actions, and that this reputation was important to the overall strength of the hospital.

Stroke has traditionally been regarded as a nonemergency problem by healthcare providers, because until recently no imme-

diate treatment had been proven effective in changing the outcome. The standard treatment has been to ensure the comfort and
safety of the victim, evaluate the extent of the damage, and to start
rehabilitation as soon as practical.

Dr. Smith is familiar with the history of the use of tPA, both
for heart attack, which was its first application, and in the recent
clinical trials for stroke. He recognized early on that accurate diagnosis of the problem is crucial to its chance of success: administration of tPA to a victim of cerebral hemorrhage, for example, would
be inappropriate and more than likely fatal to the patient.

In their discussion of the pros and cons of starting a tPA treatment program, Dr. Smith pointed out to the administrator that it
was necessary not only to have an accurate diagnosis, but that
administration of the drug must occur within three hours of the
stroke or its effectiveness would be severely reduced.

Together they identified the people who would have to understand and act swiftly. They agreed that if the new approach is to
make a difference in outcome, a major change in mind-set toward
treatment of ischemic stroke will be necessary among all hospital
personnel who will be involved. Moreover, and of particularly great
importance, it will be necessary to get area primary care physicians,
paramedics, and other emergency transportation personnel to
regard stroke as an emergency situation where time is of the
essence in diagnosis and the commencement of treatment. They
even considered the potential value of educating the general public about what would be involved.

"I don't want to mislead you, John," said the doctor. "Not only
will we have a massive education job to do, but some aspects of it
will probably have to be redone in just a few years."

"Why is that?" queried the executive.

"Because tPA is not the last word in stroke drug therapy. Sooner
or later, our protocol is bound to change again," replied Smith.

Jones pondered this point for a moment and then said, "Well,
it seems to me we will inevitably have to learn how to do things
like this on a regular basis, and now is as good a time as any. What
we learn with the program you propose will certainly be useful in

| PHASE I PLANNING |
| --- |
| Step 1: Organizing the Project |
| Step 2: Identifying Best Practitioners |
| Step 3: Preparing to Collect Data |

**PHASE I PLANNING**

**Step 1:**
Organizing
the Project

**Step 2:**
Identifying Best
Practitioners

**Step 3:**
Preparing to
Collect Data

this world of rapid change." Almost to himself he muttered, "Here we are putting portable defibrillators into the ambulances." Then, "But what about cost? Can we get it past the HMOs?"

"We won't know until we try, will we?" asked Smith. "I think a cost analysis has to be an integral part of the program."

So it was decided that they would propose an Ischemic Stroke Therapy Initiative at the next meeting of the Medical Center Executive Committee, of which Dr. Smith was a member.

The doctor gave a lot of thought as to how he would approach his Executive Committee colleagues. He ended up emphasizing why Mercy Hospital should want to embark on a stroke initiative. His argument first addressed public service to the community through improved patient outcomes, citing the enormous cost to society (over $30 billion annually) of acute care, rehabilitation, and lost productivity. He then discussed the importance of maintaining the position of preeminence enjoyed by the hospital, pointing out that the stroke initiative would add to Mercy's ability to differentiate itself in an increasingly competitive marketplace. He closed with the obvious point that prestige is a form of advertising, directly linked to continuing financial strength. Following questions about the FDA approval status of the new therapy, and some other discussion, the Committee approved a more detailed look at Dr. Smith's idea.

During the next two months, the proposed initiative was studied by a subcommittee of the Executive Committee and then discussed with the Hospital's Board of Trustees. It was finally given the go-ahead with the understanding that Dr. Smith would be overall director of the program.

## THE STORY

At the next meeting of the Executive Committee, at which he publicly accepted the stroke initiative leadership assignment, Dr. Smith summed up his understanding of the nature of the challenge in this comment to his fellow Executive Committee members:

*Our biggest job will be to convince everyone involved that a stroke is a true emergency — it's like a heart attack, where you are racing the clock the whole way. Right now, I freely admit that I don't know exactly how we're going to do this.*

PHASE I
PLANNING

Step 1:
Organizing
the Project

Step 2:
Identifying Best
Practitioners

Step 3:
Preparing to
Collect Data

After the meeting, Dr. Smith fell into conversation with the hospital's Quality Officer, Diane Turiano. Ms. Turiano, herself an RN with substantial experience as an OR nurse, had resonated strongly to her colleague's recognition that a lot of different kinds of people were going to have to change the way they thought about a suspected ischemic stroke.

Now, she said, "Charlie, when you know what you want to do and don't know how to do it, it seems to me this is exactly when you should consider a benchmarking project." Dr. Smith had considerable confidence in Ms. Turiano's good sense, and he knew just enough about benchmarking to understand her point. His immediate response was to pull out his calendar and set up a time with her when they could discuss how to structure such a project.

At their meeting, the Quality Officer gave a copy of a benchmarking book to Dr. Smith, and recommended that he pay particular attention to the section on the choice of benchmarking partners. She pointed out that the challenges in changing mindsets is not a problem confined to healthcare, and that Dr. Smith should consider what can be learned from organizations outside medicine, as well as from peer groups with relevant experience.

In a few days Dr. Smith E-mailed to Ms. Turiano a draft description for a benchmarking project, with indications where he felt he might need her help. Her reply included acceptance of her role as advisor/facilitator plus a few suggestions for strengthening the project. After one more short-turnaround iteration, they agreed that Dr. Smith should present their idea for a benchmarking project at the next regularly scheduled Executive Committee meeting on July 9, to enlist the understanding and support of the members. Ms. Turiano agreed to be ready to chime in if any of the questions seemed to need her input.

PHASE I
PLANNING

Step 1:
Organizing
the Project

Step 2:
Identifying Best
Practitioners

Step 3:
Preparing to
Collect Data

Prior to the meeting, Smith and Turiano also prepared a list of possible leaders for the stroke initiative benchmarking team. Dr. Smith naturally felt that someone from his own Emergency Medicine Department would be most appropriate, but both he and Ms. Turiano recognized that others might not agree. Specifically, both the Radiology Department, where a CT scan to rule out a cerebral hemorrhage is an essential preliminary to establishing candidacy for tPA treatment, and the nursing supervisory staff, who must manage and carry out the new stroke protocol, might each want to provide the team leader. So one from each of these groups was included on the list, four in all.

Dr. Smith's presentation was very brief and went well. It followed the outline in the prereading material he had distributed to the other members of the Executive Committee (Figure 1).

**Figure 1. Executive Committee presentation, July 9, 1996.**

Proposed Benchmarking Project in Support of the Ischemic Stroke Therapy Initiative Program

- Purpose: To identify the best available method for implementing a major change in the initial stages of treatment of suspected ischemic stroke
- Proposed approach: Benchmarking of major changeover processes in healthcare and non-healthcare settings
- Resource requirements (Estimate)
  - Team leader: 1 person, up to 1/2 time
  - Nursing : 1 person, up to 1/4 time
  - Transportation: 1 person, up to 1/4 time
  - Radiology: 1 person, up to 1/4 time
  - House staff: 1 person, up to 1/4 time
  - Emergency Department: 1 or 2 persons, up to 1/4 time
  - Pharmacy: 1 person, up to 1/4 time
- Project duration (Estimate)—2 months

*Note:* This list of participants in the benchmarking project is representative, but is by no means the only possible one. For a discussion of team roster construction, see Part 1—Chapter 1.

Audience discussion of his presentation focused on three questions:

- What kind of reaction are you getting from the insurers?
- What do you expect by way of support for the benchmarking project, and how soon will you need it?
- How do you propose to identify possible benchmarking partners outside of healthcare?

The first question was very awkward. It was not part of the benchmarking discussion, which was the announced subject, but it was central to the stroke initiative itself and could not be brushed aside.

Diane Turiano, in her role as Quality Officer, saved the day by calling for a **process check**, pointing out that the question was relevant and legitimate in the right context, but that there was nothing useful to be gained by talking about it prematurely. Better to stick to the meeting's agenda today and schedule discussion of this issue for a later time. The suggestion was accepted by the attendees with tolerably good humor after Dr. Smith promised to return in two weeks with a description of the approach he planned to take with the HMOs. He also offered to review the status of his overall plan for starting the Ischemic Stroke Therapy Initiative.

> *Note: This case study is about a benchmarking project as seen from the point of view of its sponsor. It might therefore be claimed that no further mention of the overall plan or of the cost issue with the insurers is required. However, anyone who has responsibility for a major program in which a benchmarking project is only a part will soon discover the value of keeping the benchmarking team apprised of the full context in which their work is being done. Accordingly, a discussion of Dr. Smith's overall plan and how he handled the cost question is included in the Addendum as background for some of his later communication with the benchmarking team.*

Smith was fully prepared for the second question, of course, and diplomatically referred attendees to the project proposal that he had sent them as prereading material, where they would find a list

| PHASE I PLANNING |
| --- |
| Step 1: Organizing the Project |
| Step 2: Identifying Best Practitioners |
| Step 3: Preparing to Collect Data |

PHASE I
PLANNING

Step 1:
Organizing
the Project

Step 2:
Identifying Best
Practitioners

Step 3:
Preparing to
Collect Data

of needed participants and an estimate of the project's schedule of activities.

He also was very candid about the fact that the amount of participant's time required was only an estimate, and that the benchmarking project team would almost certainly be changing it when they got into the detailed project work planning. He was at pains to reassure them that he would personally review the benchmarking team's proposed resource requirements in the course of issuing the "**Team Charter**" to be sure that they did not go beyond what the Executive Committee was being asked to authorize. He explained in some detail that the charter was essentially a contract protecting both parties: the team knows what they are expected to deliver, and the **sponsor** (in this case, himself) knows how much it will cost in the way of resources.

Dr. Smith's reputation as an honest broker was already firmly established with his peers, so that part of the discussion went smoothly. For this reason, also, the committee saw no reason why he should not select someone from his own department to lead the team, and left the choice up to him.

The third question — about getting benchmarking partners from outside healthcare — was the one he was hoping for. He needed some ideas and he knew instinctively that if he could get his colleagues to help him flesh out this part of his plan, it would be a better plan. And, just as importantly, it would now become their plan to some degree as well.

So his reply to the question about how to find help from outside healthcare was, "Not a clue right now. Do any of you have thoughts on this?"

His candor disarmed potential critics, and the outcome of the ensuing discussion was that several contacts were suggested, two of whom were already serving on the hospital Board of Trustees. Since the hospital CEO and two other members of the Executive Committee were also members of the hospital board, they agreed to help make the first contact.

After the meeting, which Charles and Diane both felt was a success, Dr. Smith sent an E-mail to the Directors of the Radiology and Transportation departments, to the Vice President of Nursing, and to the Medical Director in his role as director of the house officers, the latter two being also members of the Executive Committee. He summarized the agreements reached at the recent Executive Committee meeting about the formation of the benchmarking team, its objective, and its staffing level. He mentioned that the team leader would be a person from the Emergency Department, to be selected in the near future, and asked them for lists of people they might recommend from their areas as candidates for the benchmarking team. He said that suitable candidates should have broad knowledge of emergency treatment processes in their work area, enjoy the highest professional regard among their peers; be good team players, and be willing to participate.

When these lists came back (and after a phone call from the head of radiology asking for more information), Dr. Smith held two important interviews: one with Lois Kent, R.N.; and the other with Mary Leighton, a medical technician. These were the two people on his Emergency Medicine staff whom he had identified as possible benchmarking team leaders.

| PHASE I PLANNING |
| :---: |
| **Step 1: Organizing the Project** |
| Step 2: Identifying Best Practitioners |
| Step 3: Preparing to Collect Data |

---

### WHAT MAKES A GOOD TEAM LEADER

The leader of a benchmarking team must be chosen with considerable care. This person must be able to function independently without benefit of an established routine, otherwise the sponsor will end up being the *de facto* team leader. Since the leader must be what the name implies—a leader in group situations—she or he is usually a person who already has at least some supervisory experience. It is also important that the team leader be attuned to how the formal and informal management mechanisms of the organization actually work, and is not dismayed by situations involving turf, status, and the like.

---

During these interviews it became clear that Ms. Kent was the right choice. Whereas these two women were very similar in their

PHASE I
PLANNING

Step 1:
Organizing
the Project

Step 2:
Identifying Best
Practitioners

Step 3:
Preparing to
Collect Data

qualifications, Ms. Leighton was currently struggling with a situation in her personal life that left her little extra energy for an assignment as demanding as this would be.

It also turned out that Lois Kent had at least a nodding acquaintance with a number of people on the roster of potential team members provided by the department heads, and felt comfortable with the prospect of working with some of them. About others, she wasn't so sure. The initial E-mail to the executives had essentially asked for the best people in the organization, whose demands of course make them the ones least likely to be able to participate. So the list of candidates that came back was a somewhat mixed bag, as Diane Turiano had warned. She did promise to keep an eye on the team's activities.

After Ms. Kent had accepted the role of team leader, she and Dr. Smith prepared a team recruiting memo and sent it out over both signatures to a list of about 20 individuals whom they had identified as good potential benchmarking team members. In the memo they explained why a benchmarking team was forming, how each person came to be on the list, and solicited each candidate's interest in participating.

While they waited for the replies, Lois Kent studied the book on benchmarking, met twice with the Quality Officer for coaching, and made the necessary arrangements for her job backfill during temporary absences from her regular duties. Dr. Smith was very helpful in the job backfill situation, juggling assignments, and talking with people about the objectives of the study Lois was to be heading up.

The response to the recruiting memo was somewhat underwhelming. Everyone in the hospital was already very busy, and with the rumor mill seething with gossip about further staff reductions, no one, neither worker nor supervisor, was willing to admit that any spare time existed. Nevertheless, and after the doctor reminded some people of the agreements reached in the Executive Committee meeting, Lois and Dr. Smith had a team with an adequate balance of experience, enthusiasm, and organizational savvy.

The first meeting of the project team was about one hour long, and went very well. Because both sponsor and team leader were somewhat doubtful about the level of commitment they were experiencing, they did a very thorough preparation for the kickoff, and it showed in the results. Their agenda was as follows:

PHASE I
PLANNING

Step 1:
Organizing
the Project

Step 2:
Identifying Best
Practitioners

Step 3:
Preparing to
Collect Data

### Agenda

- Welcome and Project Background — C. Smith, M.D. (10 min.)
- Benchmarking Process Introduction — D. Turiano, R.N. (10 min.)
- Resources – C. Smith, M.D. (5 min.)
- Overall Project Outline — L. Kent, R.N. (5 min.)
- Discussion – ALL (25 min.)
- Next steps — L. Kent, R.N. (5 min.)

A few comments about this meeting are in order.

First, the meeting was structured to be a clear baton-passing from the sponsor to the team leader, and was intended to be one of Dr. Smith's few face-to-face encounters with the team. He would be handing over the actual running of the team to Lois Kent, and at this meeting his job as **sponsor** was to impress upon the members of the team the importance of what they were doing. He did this in his introductory remarks by simply telling the story behind the Executive Committee's decision to pioneer the new stroke treatment.

Later in the meeting he drove his point home convincingly when he talked about resources. He described the conditions of team participation: released time with job backfill, project participation as a formal job performance objective, and team training and facilitation as needed. When he mentioned that he would authorize travel for site visits if that was indicated, his audience became believers that this project really mattered to Mercy Hospital leadership.

Diane Turiano's introduction to the benchmarking process was short. She mostly spoke about Phase I — Planning, emphasizing the need for patience, saying that time spent on doing a thorough job here would be well rewarded in the end. She also spoke about the idea of working with benchmarking partners from outside healthcare, mentioning that she and Dr. Smith would be

149

PHASE I
PLANNING

Step 1:
Organizing
the Project

Step 2:
Identifying Best
Practitioners

Step 3:
Preparing to
Collect Data

providing some contacts for the team. She ended her part of the discussion by complimenting Lois Kent on her rapid assimilation of the fundamentals of benchmarking.

By the time Lois Kent got up to speak, both she and the benchmarking project had a great deal of credibility, and she got right down to business. She presented the broad outline of the project plan that had been put together so far, and said that the first job of the team was going to be the detailed project planning. She also described the idea of the team's **charter**, indicating that it would be one of their first group outputs.

She then said that she was sure the group had any number of questions about all that had been thrown at them. She noted that she would be in frequent contact with Dr. Smith and Ms. Turiano as the project proceeded, but that now was the best time to hear from them directly.

The ensuing discussion was lively, heavily repetitive (questions about release time, for example, kept coming up in various guises), but worthwhile.

The meeting closed with a brief housekeeping discussion. The time of the next meeting was set, and the team members learned that their permanent meeting place would be the Internal Medicine Department conference room, a very prestigious location. They departed with much to think about.

True to his word, Dr. Smith shared his cost/benefit analysis of the stroke initiative (see Addendum) with his colleagues on the Executive Committee at its meeting on July 23. He told them he was scheduled to meet on July 30 with the COO of the largest HMO in the area, the first of three such meetings. They wished him the best of success.

The next key event in the benchmarking project, as seen from Dr. Smith's perspective, was recruitment of two benchmarking partners from outside healthcare. This was accomplished via a pair of meetings that he and Diane Turiano held with two local business people. One was on July 24, with Jack Scott, a member of the hospital's Board of Trustees and local Division Manager for a huge multinational corporation. The other was on July 26, with Pierre Jacob, founder and CEO of a major local business firm. (Contact with Mr. Jacob was made through an attorney on the Board of Trustees.)

The two meetings were very similar in tone and outcome. In both instances, Smith and Turiano followed a game plan they had worked out beforehand:

After introductions and pleasantries, the doctor described in lay terms the Ischemic Stroke Therapy Initiative and its place in Mercy Hospital's vision of providing continuing improvement in cost-effective healthcare and the quality of life in the local ommunity. He provided some illustrative figures on the avoided costs of rehabilitation if the new treatment were used successfully.

Diane then explained how the mind-set of providers toward stroke treatment would have to change in order for the new treatment to be used, and the need for a benchmarking project to learn how to bring this change about. She expressed the belief that the stroke initiative team could learn a lot from industry about how to deploy a major process change in a large, diversified, and geographically spread out workforce.

Smith and Turiano counted on the idea that both businessmen would be flattered and would agree to help. They were right.

The outcome of the meeting with Mr. Scott is documented in a letter to him recording the agreements reached at the meeting in his office (see Figure 2). A similar letter was sent to Mr. Jacob.

Next Dr. Smith tackled the head of the largest local HMO, armed with his cost/benefit analysis (see Addendum). He was joined in this discussion by Henry Moore, the hospital's CFO, and Joe Wilson, the systems analyst who was intimately familiar with the data and the analytical methodology. Preparation for the meeting was along the same lines as that for the meetings with Scott and Jacob, the business executives.

The meeting took place on July 30, and was another success. The HMO executive agreed to have his actuaries and marketing people work with Mr. Wilson and the Mercy Finance Department to validate the cost projections for the HMO subscriber population. He said that the HMO would come on board for a one-year trial period if the projections worked out. It was not lost on the

| PHASE I PLANNING |
| :---: |
| Step 1: Organizing the Project |
| Step 2: Identifying Best Practitioners |
| Step 3: Preparing to Collect Data |

PHASE I
PLANNING

Step 1:
Organizing
the Project

Step 2:
Identifying Best
Practitioners

Step 3:
Preparing to
Collect Data

HMO executive that there was significant marketing value for the HMO if it announced the addition of a promising new treatment for a prevalent disease to its list of covered benefits, and without an increase in subscriber premium payment. He was privately skeptical of some of Dr. Smith's assumptions, particularly the one about the provider service differential between neurologists and PCPs, but he felt the overall cost exposure would not be excessive, considering the projected benefits.

---

**Figure 2. Letter to Mr. J. Scott.**

July 25, 1996
Mr. Jack Scott, Division Vice President
XYZ Corporation
100 Broadway
New Holland, NY 10001

Dear Mr. Scott:

Thank you very much for the opportunity to discuss with you on July 24 the Ischemic Stroke Therapy Initiative at Mercy Hospital, and for your generous offer of assistance to our benchmarking project connected with this initiative.

Our understanding of the agreements reached in our meeting are as follows:

1. XYZ Corporation will respond to a questionnaire to be developed by our benchmarking team. Estimated time to complete: under three hours.

2. XYZ Corporation will host a site visit, should it become desirable, by members of our benchmarking team either here in New Holland or at corporate headquarters in Center City, NJ. Estimated visit time: no more than one day during regular business hours.

3. Subject matter to be covered is limited to the approaches used by XYZ to assure successful introduction of major new business processes simultaneously into different parts of the organization, and in different locations. No proprietary information will be discussed.

4. Mercy Hospital's contact within XYZ is to be Ms. Janet Seeley, Manager, Business Process Development, telephone 111-2222. You will inform her of our request, and Lois Kent, the Mercy Hospital benchmarking team leader, will call her in a few days to begin work.

We also wish to thank you for your suggestion that we involve people from the hospital with a communications background in our benchmarking effort. We intend to follow up on that suggestions as soon as possible.

Very truly yours,

Charles Smith, M.D.
Diane Turiano, R.N.

---

The actuarial, legal, and financial paperwork associated with the agreements reached were handled by the appropriate administrative units in the hospital and need not concern us further here.

On August 5, a few days after this series of meetings, Dr. Smith met with Lois Kent and told her of his success in obtaining offers of help. She was duly grateful, but wondered out loud whether the two companies proposed were the best in the world at the task of rolling out a major new business process. Charles's rejoinder was that he had discussed this point with Diane Turiano, and they had ended up agreeing that the object of benchmarking is to do a better job by being better informed, and that you can learn from anyone who knows more than you do. Moreover, both of the businesses involved were already known to be fast-moving and innovative, so they were probably in the upper quartile of performance in the area in question. He and Lois ended up agreeing that, for their purposes, and in their state of knowledge, using well-qualified contacts who were immediately available had many practical advantages over a search for the "best of the best," however desirable that might be, theoretically.

Next, the doctor described some advice he had gotten from Jack Scott about involving people with experience in communicating new things to the workforce, and they discussed briefly who that might be at Mercy. It was decided that this was a good topic for the team to chew on. (The team later chose Mary Baldwin of the Marketing Department, because of her knowledge of the "big-picture" strategy at Mercy, her network of contacts within administration and elsewhere in the institution, and her feel for how to sell an idea. Dr. Smith arranged for her to join the team, promptly notifying the Executive Committee of this move.)

Lois then showed Dr. Smith a draft of a team charter that she had developed with her team. After studying it he asked her to make one major change — specifically, to expand the scope of the project to include a process for educating the front-line people at the participating HMOs regarding the new stroke initiative. He described to Lois the meetings he had held with key executives at the HMOs, and explained that they had stressed that the sub-

| PHASE I PLANNING |
|---|
| Step 1: Organizing the Project |
| Step 2: Identifying Best Practitioners |
| Step 3: Preparing to Collect Data |

PHASE I
PLANNING

Step 1:
Organizing
the Project

Step 2:
Identifying Best
Practitioners

Step 3:
Preparing to
Collect Data

scriber-contact people must understand the new game plan in order to make the changeover as smooth as possible.

After this change, Charles and Lois agreed to issue the charter jointly, saying that it should be read into the minutes of the next team meeting. Figure 3: Team Charter.

**Figure 3. Benchmarking team charter.**

This charter records our agreement that a project team will benchmark methods of successfully introducing major new work processes in a system with many interacting professional specialties distributed across several organizations and many physical locations. The project is in support of the Mercy Hospital Ischemic Stroke Therapy Initiative.

The team will be composed of the following individuals:

Daniel Clark, RT, Supervisor — Radiology Department

Sue Sprite, R.N., Supervisor — Surgery Department

Mary Baldwin, Manager — Marketing Department (as of 8/9/96)

William Trask, Manager — Transportation Department

Raj Mukerjee, M.D. — Emergency Medicine Department (house staff)

Willis Chambers, PhM — Supervisor, Pharmacy

Lois Kent, R.N. — Team Leader, Emergency Medicine Department

Team members will spend up to one-fourth time on the project, for a period of six weeks beginning July 22, 1996. The team leader will spend up to half-time. The project final report and recommendations are due on or before September 3, 1996.

If there is demonstrated need, up to six person-days of off-campus travel is authorized.

The Project Work Plan is outlined on Attachment 1. It may be subject to later modification.

The project will address the following requirements:

1. Identify the best available approach to achieving the following objective:

   To introduce a new protocol for suspected ischemic stroke in which all providers of medical services and ancillary services are motivated to treat the situation as an emergency in which very rapid and accurate diagnosis of the patient's condition is critically important to the patient's recovery.

2. Prepare recommendations for a plan to achieve the objective that addresses how primary-care physicians, paramedics, ambulance

154

drivers, Emergency Department personnel, Radiology Department personnel, and certain HMO personnel are to be educated about their roles in administering the new protocol. Recommendations are to include explicit statements about how best to adapt recommended procedures that are not presently in use in a healthcare setting.

3. Make recommendations concerning other actions discovered in the course of the benchmarking study that could assist in achieving the objective.

Charles Smith, M.D.
Lois Kent, R.N.
August 5, 1996

| PHASE I PLANNING |
|---|
| Step 1: Organizing the Project |
| Step 2: Identifying Best Practitioners |
| Step 3: Preparing to Collect Data |

## Attachment 1 – Project Work Plan

| | |
|---|---|
| week 1 (7/22/96) | Prepare list of potential benchmarking partners drawn from healthcare organizations<br>– Discuss contents of questionnaire |
| week 2 (7/29/96) | Identify screener questions<br>– Contact potential partners with screener<br>– Prepare first draft of questionnaire |
| week 3 (8/5/96) | Pilot questionnaire internally<br>– Finalize questionnaire<br>– Mail questionnaire |
| week 4 (8/12/96) | Compile questionnaire results<br>– Identify site visit issues<br>– Schedule site visits |
| week 5 (8/19/96) | Site visits<br>– Draft recommendations |
| week 6 (8/26/96) | Sell recommendations internally<br>– Finalize recommendations |
| 9/3/96 | – FINAL REPORT DUE |
| TBD | Presentation to Executive Committee |

At the next meeting of the Executive Committee on August 6, Dr. Smith briefly filled his colleagues in on what they already knew via the grapevine, namely, that the major HMOs supported the Ischemic Stroke Initiative in principle. He said that the benchmarking team was in full swing, their charter having been formally issued just the day before. He also asked for 10 minutes on the agenda at the next meeting for an update on team progress.

PHASE I
PLANNING

Step 1:
Organizing
the Project

Step 2:
Identifying Best
Practitioners

Step 3:
Preparing to
Collect Data

He might not have done this if he had known what next week had in store for him.

What happened was that the benchmarking team had begun thinking about what kinds of questions they would ask their benchmarking partners in healthcare. Not knowing that another group was already working along related lines (see Addendum), the team lost sight of its charter and began to speculate about what the new protocol would look like. They had gone so far as to do process flow-charting of how Mercy currently handles suspected AMI cases (also time-urgent emergencies), identified measurements of AMI treatment process quality, and developed a "strawman" proposed process for stroke victims based on this model. Having identified areas of dissatisfaction with their "strawman," the team now felt that they knew what to ask the other hospitals about. In short, they were out in left field, well along in doing the work of one of the other projects in the overall stroke initiative program.

Charles Smith learned of all this in a hallway conversation with Lois, where he asked her casually,

"How are things going in the big project, Lois?"

He was on the way to a consult, but her enthusiastic response stopped him in his tracks. He listened with mounting dismay as she talked excitedly about the latest team activities. The doctor finally asked Lois if she could stop by his office later that day. He went off down the hall, thoughtfully, sipping his coffee.

By the time they met, the doctor had decided he would let Lois down gently (because her mistake was from an excess of zeal) and then get the team back on the track. This he did, gracefully accepting the responsibility for not making clear to the team how their work fit into the bigger picture. Together they figured that the team had probably lost a week, but maybe they could make it up.

On August 20, Dr. Smith summarized for the Executive Committee the chartered activities to date of his benchmarking team. He first described their successful search for good benchmarking partners, which now included two other tertiary-care

156

teaching hospitals with a strong reputation for innovation in treatment protocols, as well as the two non-healthcare businesses.

He next described the measurements that the team intended to use to identify the most effective processes for rolling out a new protocol — things like percent of those with a need to know who receive and understand the message within the scheduled time. Then he explained the development of the questionnaire that the team would use in their interaction with the other institutions. Using sample questions from the questionnaire, he illustrated how the team hoped to discover the best approach to communicating the new stroke protocol to PCPs, Mercy Hospital ER and radiology personnel, medical transport company personnel, nursing home personnel, and the front-line people at the participating HMOs.

He closed by mentioning his decision to authorize travel for site visits to two locations: one of the teaching hospitals, and a branch of the large multinational corporation. He explained how the team had arrived at their choice of sites to visit, and said that he was convinced it would be money well spent. Travel to the local business's site would involve no travel cost, of course. The site visits were scheduled to take place during the next three days.

At the very end he acknowledged that he thought the team might miss its deadline by a week or so, but the improvement in the output would be worth the inconvenience. In the interest of avoiding extraneous detail, he made no mention of the charter scope problem to this group. (He did, however, discuss it with Diane Truriano, as a **lesson-learned** that she should add to her fund of knowledge.)

Dr. Smith attended the regular 8:00 A.M. Monday meeting of the benchmarking team on August 26. Lois Kent had told him on the preceding Friday that the team planned to work through the weekend going over their findings at the site visits, comparing them with what the questionnaires had revealed, and, hopefully, developing their action recommendations.

By now the other major developmental parts of the stroke initiative program were largely completed, and Dr. Smith was anxious to roll it out in actual practice. The benchmarking team's job was

**PHASE I PLANNING**

Step 1: Organizing the Project

Step 2: Identifying Best Practitioners

Step 3: Preparing to Collect Data

to tell him how best to do that, and he was eager to hear their recommendations.

From the doctor's point of view, the meeting was a disappointment. He found a team that was full of enthusiasm, clearly pleased with what they had found out, but without a set of recommendations. The problem: undigested input.

What the team needed and asked for was more time. They said that they needed time to be sure they had found the right set of procedures for educating the various groups who would be involved in using the new emergency protocol. The team members, sometimes all talking at once, described how they had learned some very interesting things from the other teaching hospital about how to bring the radiologists and ambulance drivers on board, but they had learned some equally valuable things from the local business firm that they thought would be most applicable to the education of the HMO folks. And they had acquired all sorts of neat ideas about how to talk to the PCPs, who everyone agreed were central to the whole program. They weren't sure, however, how it all fit together. Most importantly, they had not talked to anyone in the hospital about the practicalities of putting their findings to work. As the representative from the pharmacy put it, "Until we can convert our good findings into recommendations for specific action by a specific department, we haven't really completed our job, have we?" So they needed about another week, assuming they could have access to the right people.

> **PHASE III**
> **INTEGRATION**
>
> **Step 8:**
> **Communicating**
> **the Results**
>
> **Step 9:**
> **Establishing**
> **Goals**

During the hubbub (which fortunately helped Dr. Smith conceal his disappointment), Diane Turiano, the Quality Officer, walked in. She had been invited via a Sunday night telephone call from Lois Kent, and had been able to leave her scheduled meeting early to attend this session. Her immediate reaction was to pick up a marker and turn to the ubiquitous flip-chart.

"Let's list the things that are settled right now, the things you all agree you want to do and know how to do," said Diane. The team had little difficulty in identifying these, and Diane wrote them on the chart.

"Now," she said, "let's list the things that are still up in the air, indicating which are the ones you aren't even sure you want to do, and which are the ones you know you want, but aren't sure who should be involved in doing them."

The first item that surfaced was the question of how to handle contact with nurse-practitioners. One of the hospital benchmarking partners had alerted the team to the growing importance of these providers in rural areas, and had convinced them of the need to give them information very similar to what would be provided to the primary-care physicians. The problem was that they were not sure who to approach at Mercy to get this job done. Diane's response was to write this issue on the chart, then ask for other problems.

With this and other similar helpful actions, Diane focused the group on organizing their material and thoughts. When it became clear that progress was back on track, Smith left as unobtrusively as possible, giving an OK sign to Lois when he reached the door. Later that day she validated the team's estimate of another week's work, provided they could have strong planning support from the Marketing and Community Relations Departments. Dr. Smith agreed to the request for more time and promised to talk to the people whose help was needed.

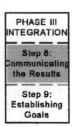

Everyone did what they said they would do. Dr. Smith paved the way for the needed support, and the team delivered their recommendations to Dr. Smith in a meeting on September 9, just one week after the original deadline (see Figure 4).

These recommendations, which were rather detailed, showed clearly that a lot more work remained to be done. After much clarifying discussion and probing of alternatives, Dr. Smith felt he understood the recommendations, accepted them, and announced his intention to present them at the next meeting of the hospital's Executive Committee.

He invited the entire benchmarking team to attend during his portion of this meeting, and publicly thanked them for their contribution during his presentation.

**Figure 4. Benchmarking team recommendations.**

1. Be sure that everyone who will be affected by or involved in carrying out the Ischemic Stroke Therapy Initiative (ISTI) is given *at least as much* information as they will need to perform their function. All members of every group involved in carrying out the new stroke protocol should be provided with the same basic package of information. It should include:

   - Cover letter from Dr. Smith and John Jones, Mercy Hospital CEO, with a summary description of the Ischemic Stroke Therapy Initiative and its rationale.

   - Letters from HMOs with expression of support and cooperation.

   - Description of ideal sequence of events when a suspected ischemic stroke alert occurs, beginning with initial telephone call and ending with patient admitted and stabilized. (To be supplied by the ISTI Protocol Development project)

   - Brief description of steps being taken to educate other groups who will be involved (in-service training for ED personnel at Mercy Hospital, etc.)

2. Be sure that everyone in the chain of providers is given the same work process information.

3. Announce up front the training schedule for all people who will be involved in carrying out some portion of the new protocol. Get started on preparation of the training materials ASAP.

4. Tailor supplementary communications to the individual subpopulations involved, but without losing sight of recommendation #2. Specifically:

   - For members of the Emergency Department and Radiology Department of Mercy Hospital: provide a letter announcing the schedule of in-service training in the new stroke treatment

   — For physicians with admitting privileges at Mercy Hospital, particularly the Primary Care Physicians: provide copies of appropriate journal articles (e.g., NEJM *333*, 1581 - 1587 (1995)) regarding clinical experience with the effectiveness of the new tPA protocol.

   - For owners and/or managers of medical transportation services companies: provide a letter describing their role in the ISTI and seeking their cooperation in educating ambulance drivers and paramedics in the new protocol. Letter is to be accompanied by a supply of information packets that will provide summary references to medical literature and include specific details of what to look for upon arrival at the scene of the emergency. Letter should also announce that additional training material will be provided at the time of each person's biennial EMS recertification training.

   - For insurers, HMOs and third-party administrators:
   provide a letter to the Chief Operating Officer announcing the ISTI and asking for cooperation in informing and training their front-line physi-

cian-contact and subscriber-contact personnel. Included with letter should be a supply of information packets for contact employees containing a description of the ISTI, with summary references to medical literature and including specific details of what paramedics will be looking for upon arrival at the scene of the emergency.

– For nursing /assisted-living home administrators:
provide a personalized cover letter describing the ISTI initiative, plus specific details of what to look for if they suspect one of their patients is suffering from a stroke. The letter should mention that Mercy Hospital people will be available to provide nursing staff training upon request.

In addition, a letter should be sent to *every* M.D. in the Mercy Hospital catchment area, to the Emergency Department heads in all area hospitals, and to all the independent radiology practices announcing the ISTI with minimal detail. (This may seem like overkill, but the object is to build a solid base of informed peers who will be more likely to support the ISTI if they know what it is about.)

5. Schedule the dissemination of information packages in the following time sequence: Mercy Hospital ED, Mercy Hospital Radiology Department, other hospitals' ED personnel, Mercy Hospital general population, non-Mercy professional providers, HMOs, medical transportation services companies, nursing homes, subscribers, media. Coordinate the physical appearance of all information packets with a distinctive look. It is recognized that the media will learn of the ISTI well in advance of the desired time in the sequence. A bare-bones package should be prepared for when this occurs, with promise of a story containing full details by a specified date. See also recommendation #8 below.

6. For all activities involving use of computers (e.g., computers used in support of telephone conversations by HMO subscriber- and provider-contact personnel), be sure that adequate training is provided, and that help screens and a help desk are up and running well ahead of first on-line use.

7. Do not involve independent radiology groups (except for basic information packet) until after an initial pilot of the ISTI in the Mercy Hospital Radiology Department.

8. Communication to the community has two parts:

   a. Subscriber communication: This activity should be planned and carried out by the individual HMOs with technical support from the ISTI program.

   b. Media communication: This activity should be planned and carried out by the Mercy Hospital Community Relations Department with technical support from the ISTI program.

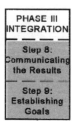

PHASE III
INTEGRATION

Step 8:
Communicating
the Results

Step 9:
Establishing
Goals

---

Fortunately, the master timetable for the whole ischemic stroke program had allowed two months to carry out the actions recommended by the benchmarking team before its scheduled rollout on

November 1. So now it was a matter of completing the detailed planning and doing the work.

This planning was done in close cooperation with the Marketing and Communications Departments, and went very smoothly, with minimal attention from Dr. Smith. By bringing them into the preparation of the recommendations, the benchmarking team had begun the process of transferring ownership of the planned activities to the departments who would bear the brunt of the work effort. Accordingly, the detailed plan was generated by people who understood its context and was very practical. All the necessary communications, information packets, etc., were produced with a minimum of difficulty.

A few days before November 1, Dr. Smith and Mr. Jones met to finalize their joint letter announcing the Ischemic Stroke Therapy Initiative. Both men were in a reflective frame of mind, knowing that the real tests of the initiative were about to begin.

"Charlie," said the administrator, "the next year is going to be pretty interesting with this stroke thing. Have you thought about what you might do to keep a sort of log of what happens? I recall that we agreed that one of the reasons for undertaking the whole project was that it would give us additional experience in managing change at the system level. I think we might benefit from a record of that experience, both the good and the not-so-great. What do you think?"

"For once I'm ahead of you, John," answered the doctor. "I have already asked all three of my teams to monitor our new processes and their results. The benchmarking team has a name for it, I discovered. They call it 'lessons-learned' and it's a fairly standard practice in the Quality movement, I'm told." Then, with a wry grin, "Had occasion to use it myself, truth to tell."

"Great! Why don't we accumulate some data on how it is going — improved rehabilitation rates, how the costs compare, provider workforce disruption during the startup transient — that sort of thing. I should think the Board of Trustees would be very much interested in what we are finding out. Would you be willing to provide a briefing for them in six months or so?"

PHASE IV
ACTION

Step 10:
Developing
Action Plans

Step 11:
Implementing
the Plan/
Monitoring
Results

Step 12:
Revisiting the
Subject

162

"Of course," said Dr. Smith. "It seems to me we almost have an obligation to share our experience with our professional colleagues. And," he said, smiling, "I don't suppose the trustees would object to being the first to find out about it."

So that is what they did.

# ADDENDUM

## OVERALL STRUCTURE OF THE ISCHEMIC STROKE THERAPY INITIATIVE PROGRAM

The program comprised three major pieces:

1. Development of a detailed treatment protocol using the current approach to emergency treatment of suspected acute heart attack (AMI) as a departure point. A small task force of veteran clinicians was given this responsibility. The task force worked through professional contacts and networks, including the Stroke Center Network of the National Stroke Association. (As pointed out in Chapter 1, networks such as this are a major advantage enjoyed by the healthcare sector in benchmarking activities.)

2. The benchmarking project, with a team responsible for recommending the best way to educate and motivate everyone who might be using the new stroke protocol.

3. Negotiations with the insurance/HMO organizations involved. This portion of the work Dr. Smith undertook as his own direct responsibility after consultation with the hospital's CEO and CFO. All three agreed that these negotiations would be driven primarily by cost considerations.

## COST JUSTIFICATION FOR THE STROKE INITIATIVE

Dr. Smith knew that his approach to the HMOs would require a full cost justification, which took him straight to the hospital's

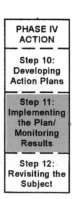

PHASE IV
ACTION

Step 10:
Developing
Action Plans

Step 11:
Implementing
the Plan/
Monitoring
Results

Step 12:
Revisiting the
Subject

Information Systems Department. Together, he and Joe Wilson, the systems analyst, developed an analysis based on the following parts:

1. First, they gathered together information about the total number of patients with suspected stroke who entered the hospital each year, noting both those who were brought in by ambulance and those who were not. Of those who were brought in by ambulance, they noted the fraction who were given full emergency treatment. They also noted the number of suspected strokes that turned out indeed to be so, and which fraction of these were diagnosed to be ischemic. (Mercy's experience was very near the national average obtained from the DRG data base: 82% ischemic vs. the national average of 80%.)

   These data gave them a basis for estimating the minimum number of cases that would be eligible for use of, and potential benefit from, the new tPA therapy.

2. Next they identified and estimated all of the costs that were allocated in the hospital's cost accounting system to the various uses of emergency services and to the same services on a nonemergency basis. (Some educated guesswork was required here.) These included first-aid actions by the paramedics and ambulance crews, reception in the ED, radiological tests, and other differences in patient treatment procedures prior to admission.

3. They then did the same thing for hospital services after admission. This was the heart of the analysis. It included the cost/day of LOS and of Physical Therapy sessions, both of which would be less for patients who had benefited from the new therapy, favoring the proposed new treatment. Offsetting these cost reductions would be the extra cost of the new drug (a major item), the extra monitoring attending its use, and the higher cost of care by specialists in neurology vs. primary-care physicians.

4. They combined all this information into a decision tree, and using standard decision analysis methodology, calculated the expected cost outcomes for the two cases: the decision to treat a suspected stroke as an emergency and the decision not to. The results were not strikingly different. In fact, they were a toss-up, within the limits of accuracy of the figures used in the analysis.

5. Finally, Dr. Smith used the relatively sparse data available from the clinical trials to draw graphs of the profiles of loss-of-function for patients who had survived an ischemic stroke, with and without tPA treatment. To these graphs he also added gross mortality figures for the two treatment modalities. Despite the admitted noisiness of the data, the differences showed clearly the effectiveness of the new protocol.

What Dr. Smith and the analyst had accomplished was to show that there might not even be additional average costs associated with use of the new approach, but that the expected patient outcomes would be significantly better.

Mr. Wilson also applied this same methodology to the case of suspected AMI, for which there was a much larger and more accurate database reaching back many years. The results were qualitatively similar, with the costs showing the expected trend over time favoring vigorous intervention, which increased his and the doctor's confidence in the approach.

## PROJECT CHRONOLOGY

| | |
|---|---|
| 6/25/96 | Dr. Smith agrees to head Ischemic Stroke Therapy Initiative (Executive Committee meeting) |
| 7/9/96 | Benchmarking project endorsed with promised support (Execetive Committee meeting) |
| 7/11/96 | Letter to key department heads seeking names of candidates for benchmarking team |
| 7/16/96 | Recruiting letter to potential team members |

| | |
|---|---|
| 7/22/96 | Kickoff meeting of benchmarking project team |
| 7/23/96 | Dr. Smith describes how he will approach HMO (Executive Committee meeting) |
| 7/24/96 | Dr. Smith and QO meet with Jack Scott, business executive |
| 7/26/96 | Dr. Smith and QO meet with Pierre Jacob, business executive |
| 7/29/96 | Second week of benchmarking project |
| 7/30/96 | Dr. Smith and CFO meet with CEO of biggest HMO |
| 8/5/96 | Third week of benchmarking project. Smith and Lois Kent issue team charter |
| 8/6/96 | Dr. Smith sketches successful meeting with HMO. Asks for time at next meeting to brief Committee on benchmarking project progress. (Executive Committee meeting) |
| 8/12/96 | Fourth week of benchmarking project |
| 8/19/96 | Fifth week of benchmarking project |
| 8/20/96 | Dr. Smith briefs Committee on benchmarking project progress. Announces decision to authorize site visits. (Executive Committee meeting) |
| 8/26/96 | Sixth week of benchmarking project |
| 9/3/96 | BENCHMARKING PROJECT REPORT DUE |
| 9/9/96 | Benchmarking project report delivered to sponsor |

# Chapter 7

# The Cranbrook Health System's Modernization Crisis

## Top Management Perspective

*Top management includes the CEO and his or her direct reports.*
*This group makes up the Executive Committee and normally*
*includes the Chief Operating Officer, Chief Financial Officer,*
*Medical Director, and other key people in the organization.*

From the perspective of top management, a benchmarking project requires the most executive attention during the preliminary stage when the overall objective is being set and the general subject area is being defined. The actual project itself usually needs comparatively little top-level involvement. Therefore, unlike the first two case studies, this one begins with events well in advance of the benchmarking effort itself.

This case study is about how the CEO of a midsized HMO uses benchmarking as a tool to organize the rescue of his company from being swallowed up or forced to close its doors. The HMO is in urgent need of streamlining its operations, which have become seriously out of date. Complicating the situation is the sudden retirement during the study of a key executive, a founding member of the management team. The issues associated with identifying the priorities for action are clarified and strong initial action is taken as part of the selection of a subject for the benchmarking study.

Things to watch for in this case study are:

How *not* to start a benchmarking project

What the CEO discovers about his role in defining a subject for benchmarking

How identifying strategic business priorities and selecting a subject for benchmarking can be two aspects of the same thing.

How to keep a high-level group discussion of a complicated subject on track, and why such techniques may be overkill when only two people are involved.

## THE SITUATION

Mr. Joe Chatsworth is the CEO of Cranbrook Health System, a mid-sized HMO in a semirural part of a populous eastern state. Cranbrook was founded shortly after passage of the HMO Act of 1973. It was thus one of the first to be in business in its catchment area, which covers over 3,000 square miles, comprising a total population of three million persons. Mr. Chatsworth's organization currently employs about 1,300 people and has a covered population of 250,000, about an 8% market penetration. Ten other HMOs also serve this population, with a combined market share of 70%. There are 25 hospitals in the area, mostly community hospitals with fewer than 200 beds and one much larger tertiary care hospital with 550 beds.

Recently a major national player in the managed-care field had been observed doing market studies in the state. The national player had talked acquisition with all of the HMOs, including Cranbrook, with varying degrees of success. Chatsworth knew his operation would be highly attractive as a takeover, but had no interest in being acquired. He had always regarded himself as a pioneer in healthcare delivery in the area, and did not wish to step aside.

Chatsworth had been even more concerned about the fact that employers contracted to Cranbrook were beginning to complain about its unacceptably high premium rates. Some, despite long-term affiliation with Cranbrook, were even talking about shifting their business to one of the younger, more aggressive HMOs.

Chatsworth had been painfully aware that Cranbrook premiums exceed those of competitors. He had not, however, determined **how** competitors were achieving cost reductions to support the premiums they were charging, nor how he should proceed in order to become competitive with them. He was aware that many operational problems must be contributing to the lack of competitiveness of Cranbrook's premium structure, but he was unsure what to tackle first, or how to go about it.

## THE STORY

Our story begins one day when Mr. Chatsworth was sitting staring out his office window in deep thought. On his desk was a pad of yellow paper with the following brief and somewhat cryptic notations:

---

### Problem/actions

- Employers, subscribers, participating doctors, hospitals, etc., all up in arms about service, i.e., errors, payment delays, report delays, GKW.
- Board question: Why Medical Loss Ratio not improving? Why reserves not up?
- What to do?!

    a. ~~Actuarial /reinsurance strategy~~
    b. Market research/Employer relations - (is price ONLY driver?)
? — > c. Medical management
  xxx d. Provider relations (PCPs, **specialist referrals**)
    e. Hospital negotiations -
— > f. **Cost reduction**
    g.

---

Chatsworth knew he wasn't getting anywhere. Like any successful executive, he had an instinctive feel for where his problems really lay. He knew that all of his serious competitors were automating their operations as fast as they could with up-to-date networked computer systems. He envied their ability to respond to requests cost-effectively *and* to be able to analyze all aspects of the business quickly — "on-line and in real-time," as they liked to say. Chatsworth knew that he couldn't continue with his present operational configuration any longer. Moreover, he recognized that his options for change were heavily constrained by the limitations of his antiquated mainframe computer. He had to *both* modernize Cranbrook's electronic data processing *and* reorganize business operations. The real issue was not what to do but what to do first, and most of all, *how* to do it. He had to take action, and soon; the need was urgent.

He had bought desktop computers for himself and his management team and asked them to learn how to use them in preparation for directing other employees more effectively when they invested in a new EDP system. He also tried to learn, because he wanted to be a smart buyer and a good customer. The problem had been to find time for the necessary practice.

As the pioneer HMO president in the area, Chatsworth had a substantial group of admirers in the local healthcare community. In fact, the CEO of the large tertiary-care hospital in the area was a member of his Board, knew all about the problems, and was a good friend. So Joe Chatsworth, never a man to let personal pride interfere with his devotion to the best interests of Cranbrook Health System, went to ask his advice.

His friend was quick to offer sympathetic understanding, telling Chatsworth he should not suffer in silence and alone. He also made it clear that the HMO head should open the window and let the future in. His advice was to go and find out how other people have dealt with the problems of major overhaul of their operations, including significant computer systems upgrades.

When asked how to do this, his response was: "Have you ever heard of benchmarking? Only vaguely? Well, personally, I might buy a book on benchmarking and get some ideas from there. Or, you could get one of your best people to read it and tell you what to do. Of course, you might hire a consultant to sort it all out for you, and you *should* get expert help, all right, but I don't think you're at the stage yet where you know what help you need. At this point I wouldn't recommend putting the fate of your whole organization in the hands of outsiders, Joe; Cranbrook is *your* responsibility."

It so happened that Mr. Chatsworth was scheduled later that week to attend a conference on capitation and risk partitioning sponsored in part by the health benefits managers of several leading corporations, and on the airplane going down he had some undisturbed time to think. At the conference he briefly cruised the exhibitor booths, picked up a book on benchmarking, and read it on the plane coming home. Interesting stuff, but he frankly couldn't see anything magical, or even really new in it. However, he decided it would do no harm to give it a try.

The following Monday morning in his executive staff meeting, Chatsworth related to the group the substance of his conversation with the board member and his subsequent reading, and ended up asking Henry Jackson, his Chief Financial Officer, if he would be willing to learn about benchmarking and lead a study to "benchmark how to improve our operations and the computer system."

Jackson, who was really the *de facto* COO of Cranbrook, was not terribly surprised by the request. As the finance officer, he inevitably had his hand in everything that went on at Cranbrook, and the computer room manager reported to him as well. However, Jackson made it clear that he would be starting from scratch with benchmarking, and hoped that expectations were not for instant progress. His leader agreed to be patient, but reminded him that the situation was urgent.

Nothing happened.

After two weeks Chatsworth went to Jackson to find out what was holding up the parade. He found two reasons for the lack of action.

- The Cranbrook CFO was simply not up to the task. Henry Jackson was one of a handful of people who, together with

| PHASE I PLANNING |
| --- |
| Step 1: Organizing the Project |
| Step 2: Identifying Best Practitioners |
| Step 3: Preparing to Collect Data |

**PHASE I
PLANNING**

**Step 1:
Organizing
the Project**

**Step 2:
Identifying Best
Practitioners**

**Step 3:
Preparing to
Collect Data**

Chatsworth, had started Cranbrook back in the '70's — another era in healthcare. Joe and Henry had been together ever since, and Henry was getting tired. (In fact, Jackson had recently confided to his wife that he was beginning to wonder if now might be the time to think about retiring. Nothing of this had been said to Chatsworth, however.)

- Under the circumstances, Jackson's charter was too vague. As Jackson himself put it, "You said to 'benchmark how to improve our operations and the computer system.' I wouldn't know where to start, Joe. Why don't you ask me to solve world hunger?"

Chatsworth was sympathetic and patient. He suggested that Jackson bring in one of those new "professional temps" that were becoming more and more fashionable. Organizations are using lawyers, architects, even doctors in these jobs, so why not a guy to look at our office systems?

It didn't work. The temporary worker, who was a person with impressive credentials and behavior to match, left after a week, confiding to Chatsworth on the way out: "I really think you have more than one problem here. I can't get anybody to talk to me. It may be out of fear, but I think it is loyalty to Mr. Jackson. I suspect people think he is being pushed into retirement, and that I am angling to be his replacement."

This comment about Henry Jackson by the departing temp was not altogether surprising to Joe Chatsworth, who determined to approach Jackson and find out for sure which way the wind was blowing.

Over the next two weeks, Chatsworth spent a lot of time with his old and valued colleague. The outcome was a retirement package that both felt was fair and properly recognized Jackson's many contributions over the years. It came out that Jackson wanted to make a quick, clean break, turning down a transitional consulting arrangement. He even begged off on helping to recruit his successor.

After the small private retirement dinner with his colleagues on the executive committee, the night before his departure with

Mrs. Jackson on a lengthy holiday, Jackson's parting words to Chatsworth, said in the unmistakable tones of old friend to old friend, were: "Good luck in figuring out what you want to do. Remember you will have to be able to explain that to the applicants for my old job."

These words left Joe Chatsworth very thoughtful. What, indeed, *do* I want to do? Hire a new CFO (new COO, if the truth were known) to replace Henry, or split the job and have a competition, with two candidates for promotion?

In this state of mind, Mr. Chatsworth began recruiting, and it did not go well. There were plenty of candidates, but people who could do the job were wary, sensing his indecision.

Recalling Henry Jackson's parting advice, Chatsworth finally sat down and formulated a description of the vacancy left by Jackson's departure. He concluded that there were really two jobs; a Chief Operating Officer and a Chief Information Officer. He decided to go after the COO, who would in turn be authorized to hire a CIO of his own choosing right off the bat.

With this approach clearly in mind, Chatsworth went back to recruiting, now able to be crisp about conditions. He also decided to mention the prospective benchmarking project to candidates for the COO position.

This proved to be an excellent tactic, and Chatsworth was able to attract a man named Duane Hess. Hess was young, but highly qualified in HMO work, obviously very comfortable with the desktop computer environment, and seemed to have a list of Information Systems contacts all ready to go. He also had a favorable attitude about benchmarking, having watched it in action — although he made it clear that he had no hands-on experience.

Hess came on board soon after his compensation package was finalized, and immediately sat down with Chatsworth to receive direction on how to get up to speed. Among other things, he asked about what to do about the benchmarking project. Did the CEO want to start it up with existing folks or wait till the new IS person came on board?

| PHASE I PLANNING |
| --- |
| **Step 1:** Organizing the Project |
| **Step 2:** Identifying Best Practitioners |
| **Step 3:** Preparing to Collect Data |

**PHASE I
PLANNING**

Step 1:
Organizing
the Project

Step 2:
Identifying Best
Practitioners

Step 3:
Preparing to
Collect Data

Joe Chatsworth had anticipated that this question would come up and replied:

*I think we could try a two-stage approach on the benchmarking thing. I learned the hard way that we have to define the scope of the project in order to make much progress in benchmarking. Now, you have to get acquainted with the business right away, and in the process you will automatically come up to speed on the issues. That will prepare you to work with me to prioritize the subjects the benchmarking project might go after. Two birds with one stone, you might say.*

*Meanwhile, you can be recruiting the CIO we agreed on. When that person comes on board, we can make the benchmarking project his/her first assignment. To get the project going, he or she must learn about the existing work processes, but that would have to happen anyway. So again we get two birds with one stone. What do you think, Duane?*

Hess saw the merits in this approach, and the two men discussed the pros and cons for a few minutes. An objection, for example, was that the new IS person would not know the people, and would need help in getting a team together. But once again Chatsworth and Hess both recognized that what they needed to do for the sake of benchmarking was something they would want to do anyway. That is, in order for the new IS officer to become fully effective in the organization, it was essential that personal ties be established with the Directors of Marketing & Sales, Customer Service, Insurance Operations, and Medical Management. If all of these people were named to a benchmarking steering committee, with the COO as chairman, they could help recruit the benchmarking team while getting acquainted with the new IS officer.

The upshot of their discussion was that Chatsworth and Hess agreed that the overall objective of the benchmarking project was still "to improve our operations and the computer system," and that the existing management team would select its general subject, based on their evaluation of the problems of the business. The new IS manager's first assignment would be to become the benchmarking team leader, prioritize the issues within the framework of the overall objective, and settle on a specific subject. Hess would serve as project sponsor. Meanwhile, he would get cracking on his recruiting task.

Not long after the discussion described above, Chatsworth and Hess met to go over Hess's initial findings and evaluation of the business. To start the meeting, Hess handed his boss a piece of paper on which he had listed the major categories of work processes as they might relate to the proposed benchmarking project (Figure 1).

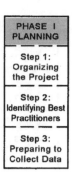

**Figure 1. Hess's list for Cranbrook Health Systems operations.**

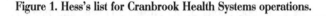

1. **Provider services database management.** Obtaining, verifying, and tracking provider data: prospecting, recruitment, contracting, credentialing and publication of the provider directories. Setting fee schedules, tracking utilization, paying claims, reporting to various governmental bodies.

2. **Employer and customer/subscriber services.** Providing employers with current data in provider directory to assist in plan selection and provider selection. Carry out enrollment, issuance of insurance ID cards, subscriber orientation, respond to subscriber questions, concerns etc.

3. **Business analysis and marketing.** Sales statistics and projections, renewals/new business/lost business. Analysis by region, group size, type of plan, account representative, month of enrollment.

4. **Operations and operations monitoring.** Claims processing, manual review, remittance preparation, check cutting and mailing.

5. **Provider Panel Management.** Maintenance of up-to-date patient lists for each PCP.

6. **Medical Management.** Monitoring and analysis of preventive services, effectiveness of disease and episode management guidelines, hospital days, professional, pharmacy and laboratory services, information timeliness for effective collaboration in chemical dependency, substance abuse and behavioral health, case management of high-risk pregnancies and other at-risk populations.

7. **Operations reporting.** Provider panel. capitation, utilization, clinical quality measures, customer/subscriber inquiries and complaints.

| PHASE I PLANNING |
| :---: |
| **Step 1:** Organizing the Project |
| **Step 2:** Identifying Best Practitioners |
| **Step 3:** Preparing to Collect Data |

Chatsworth was impressed with Hess's grasp of the operation as evidenced by the way he had organized the list. For a moment he silently congratulated himself on his excellent choice of a new COO and then said, "That's quite a list, Duane. What do you think we should go after first?"

The ensuing discussion was long and involved, and it was not confined to just one meeting. Fortunately, the two men had hit it off at the personal level from the first moment, so the exchanges were easy and informal. Each of them kept a few personal notes as they went along, but nothing elaborate was written down. They finally ended up agreeing that three areas: provider services database management; operations & operations analysis; and medical management seemed to share top priority in their minds for beginning the transition to a networked operations management system for Cranbrook. There were, thus, three possible subjects for a benchmarking project, with no obvious way to break the tie.

"So what do we do now, coach?" asked Hess after they had reached this point.

This was an easy one for Joe Chatsworth. His management style called for laying a situation out for his executive team in enough detail so that they could provide useful input when he sought their advice. So he asked Hess to prepare to do this by summarizing the things they had talked about. Chatsworth suggested that he tidy it up a bit, and explain the criteria by which they had instinctively weighed the various possibilities.

They had, for example, agreed without discussion that what they should benchmark must provide benefit to their cost picture as soon as possible. They had also recognized that, since the purpose of a benchmarking project is to guide action, and the sooner the better, they should benchmark a subject that would become the first focus of the transition to the new computer system. From this it followed that they would not want it to be too much in the public eye, because the start-up glitches would probably not be a pretty thing to watch. There were other considerations as well, and altogether Chatsworth and Hess concluded that they had about five criteria by which they had sorted and prioritized Hess's original list, albeit somewhat subconsciously.

When they were satisfied with their list of prioritization criteria, Duane commented somewhat ruefully that it might have been a good idea to develop that list first and run the various options through some sort of a decision mill, things might have gone faster. Chatsworth agreed in part, but pointed out that the utility of formal processes goes up as the group involved in the decision-making gets larger. His feeling was that the two of them had not really needed it, but that the formal approach would show major advantages when the whole management team participated.

> **PHASE I PLANNING**
>
> **Step 1:** Organizing the Project
>
> **Step 2:** Identifying Best Practitioners
>
> **Step 3:** Preparing to Collect Data

The next step was to have an executive committee meeting to lay out the situation for that group's consideration. This would be an important meeting for a number of reasons:

- The subjects to be discussed cut to the heart of the viability of the whole Cranbrook organization. This was serious business.

- Joe Chatsworth did not intend to submit to a vote the choice of what to do first in the move to office automation (which would drive the choice of subject for the benchmarking project). But he did want his executive team's input, and their enthusiastic support of the decision. Everyone at the meeting must legitimately feel that his or her contribution was making a difference.

- Also, the ill-fated first attempt at benchmarking had left a memory that had to be washed away.

- Finally, this initial assessment of the operation would be Duane Hess's first major presentation to the management group, and Chatsworth was anxious that it go well.

The meeting took place in the boardroom as usual, but not at the regularly scheduled time. Instead it was convened at noon on Wednesday, June 18, starting with lunch and running throughout the afternoon. The usual group was present: Abbie Aylesworth, Vice President for Customer Service Operations; Ben Bolt, VP of Marketing & Sales; Cindy Corbin, M.D., Medical Director; Doug Dempsey, VP Insurance Operations; Ellie Engstrom, VP Human Resources; Hess, and Chatsworth.

177

PHASE I
PLANNING

Step 1:
Organizing
the Project

Step 2:
Identifying Best
Practitioners

Step 3:
Preparing to
Collect Data

The agenda had been announced at the time the meeting was called, and it had only two items: Duane Hess's presentation of his initial observations about the needs of Cranbrook Health System, and a discussion to be led by the CEO of the priorities for action. Mr. Chatsworth had also made it clear that he wanted this to be a decision meeting, and expected that everyone would come prepared to participate vigorously.

Duane Hess was a good speaker and he had prepared very carefully, so his presentation went well. At the beginning, he spoke without notes, but when he came to the material leading up to the discussion of priorities for immediate action, he put up a transparency from which he summarized the conversations that he and Joe Chatsworth had had over the last two weeks (Table 1).

**Table 1. Duane Hess's transparency.**

| WORK PROCESS CATEGORY | A | B | C | D | E |
|---|---|---|---|---|---|
| 1. Provider services database management | M | M | M | H | H |
| 2. Employer and customer/ subscriber services | L | L | M | M | L |
| 3. Business analysis and marketing | L | H | M | M | L |
| 4. Operations and operations monitoring | H | H | M | M | H |
| 5. Provider panel management | L | H | M | H | L |
| 6. Medical management | H | H | M | L | H |
| 7. Operations reporting | L | H | M | M | L |

Decision Criteria

A. Immediate Operating Cost Reduction

B. Low Subscriber Visibility

C. Ease of Implementation

D. Low Capital Exposure

E. High Provider Concern

Hess candidly acknowledged that the slide looked much neater and better organized than the discussions that produced it, but it captured the substance pretty well. He said that the list of decision criteria accurately showed the considerations that he and the boss had agreed were most important. He explained that the letters H, M, and L indicated the judgments that they had made as to how important (H for high, etc.) these criteria were when they were applied to each of the categories of activities that made up the work of the HMO. He then indicated that very little was cast in concrete yet, and that the matrix in the slide was intended partly as a tool to help keep the discussion focused. With that he handed the meeting over to Mr. Chatsworth.

| PHASE I PLANNING |
| --- |
| Step 1: Organizing the Project |
| Step 2: Identifying Best Practitioners |
| Step 3: Preparing to Collect Data |

Joe Chatsworth was a naturally affable man, and could be charming if he chose. Today he wanted a full-bodied, free-flowing discussion, but he also wanted to reach his goal — a strongly supported consensus on the priorities for Cranbrook's transition to a more cost-effective environment. He began by saying that nothing was firmly decided yet, and he wanted everyone's candid input. He pointed out, however, that he also wanted the best possible decision. To get this, the meeting needed some ground rules.

1. Discussion about the work categories and their content is OK.
2. Challenges to the ratings (H, M, L) are OK.
3. Proposals for additions to the list of criteria are OK.
4. Discussion about the weight to be given each criterion in the decision process is OK.
5. Disagreements are OK, even encouraged, but they must be identified as being about one of the preceding four items.

Everyone agreed and they were off.

Chatsworth began the discussion by pointing out that the entries in column "C" (Ease of Implementation) on the transparency were all "M," of "medium" importance. This merely reflected the fact that neither he nor Duane felt they knew enough about the installation of computer systems to make a distinction, and had waffled. This immediately led to a question about whether it would be wise to agree on the weightings of the criteria before the group did anything else. Duane Hess said that this was

179

PHASE I
PLANNING

Step 1:
Organizing
the Project

Step 2:
Identifying Best
Practitioners

Step 3:
Preparing to
Collect Data

a good point, and he just happened to have another transparency that illustrated how weighting could be included and how it might affect the outcome of the ratings (Table 2).

Table 2. The decision matrix.

| Work Process Category | Score Equal Weighting* | Score Differential Weighting** |
|---|---|---|
| 1. Provider services database management | 12 | 27 |
| 2. Employer and customer/ subscriber services | 7 | 14 |
| 3. Business analysis and marketing | 9 | 18 |
| 4. Operations and operations monitoring | 13 | 30 |
| 5. Provider panel management | 10 | 20 |
| 6. Medical management | 12 | 28 |
| 7. Operations reporting | 9 | 18 |

* Weighting:
 H = 3; M = 2; L = 1
 A = B = C = D = E = 1

**Weighting:
 H = 3; M = 2; L = 1
 A = 3; B = 2; C = 1; D = 2; E = 3

Someone then asked why they didn't just drop criterion "C, Ease of Implementation," since it was not a useful discriminant. Hess answered that it didn't really make any difference, since all it did in this instance was to provide a uniform offset to the individual scores (this subtlety may have been lost on a few of the participants), but agreed that it simplified the number of things they had to talk about if they were to drop it. Ben Bolt, however, disagreed, pointing out that, whereas the executive group might not be able to discriminate on this point, the new Information Systems officer would certainly know, and they should keep it on the list pending that person's arrival and input. And so it went for several hours.

The outcome of the meeting was unanimous agreement that two of the major kinds of work activities at the HMO had top priority for first action:

- Operations and operations monitoring
- Medical management

Most of those present were also eager to get on with the needed changes. That feeling was not universal, to be sure, and everyone felt some uneasiness about the future. However, the discussions had brought out problems and urgencies associated with the current set-up that had never all been put on the table at once before. The atmosphere was unmistakable: we can't go on much longer doing things the way we have been. Like it or not, change was on the way.

Joe Chatsworth's wrap-up remarks were brief and gracious. He thanked everyone for their thoughtful contributions and vigorous participation in the meeting. He said quite sincerely that he believed they could not have achieved such a knowledgeable consensus any other way.

The next steps, he said, would be to get the new CIO on board as quickly as possible, get that person acquainted with the people and the operation, and begin the benchmarking project, which would be needed to guide the organization into the brave new world of networked operations.

He then announced that Susan Strickland was to be the new IS officer, and that she would show up on July 1. There was a murmur of approval at this, since everyone in the room had interviewed her and been impressed, both by her data processing credentials and by her behavior. They also knew that she did not have actual HMO experience and would need education in the specifics of their business. So when Chatsworth asked for volunteers to be on her benchmarking project steering committee, everyone raised a hand, was accepted, and the meeting ended on that note of leadership solidarity.

**PHASE I PLANNING**

**Step 1:** Organizing the Project

**Step 2:** Identifying Best Practitioners

**Step 3:** Preparing to Collect Data

<table>
<tr><td>

**PHASE I PLANNING**

**Step 1:**
Organizing
the Project

**Step 2:**
Identifying Best
Practitioners

**Step 3:**
Preparing to
Collect Data

</td></tr>
</table>

## THE BENCHMARKING PROJECT STORY

Susan Strickland reported for work on July 1. She was greeted by Duane Hess, her new boss, and shown by him to her office. After they had chatted for a few minutes about practical matters, Hess took her down the hall to where Mr. Chatsworth was waiting to greet her. It happened to be a very busy day for the CEO, so he moved swiftly through the pleasantries and got quickly to her first assignment. At the time of her interviews, they had talked about the benchmarking project, but this was prior to the June 18 meeting. Now Chatsworth briefly described the meeting, its process, and the outcome, and asked her what could be done to help her get started.

Before she could answer, he mentioned that he could get the loan of a facilitator/trainer from the large tertiary-care hospital, and he would be happy to make contacts with HMOs from other parts of the country whose executives he knew.

Ms. Strickland thanked him, accepted the offer of the facilitator help, and said that when she developed her list of potential benchmarking partners, she would definitely be back to him. She seemed particularly grateful for the establishment of the steering committee, remarking that in her experience they could be very helpful to a benchmarking activity that cut across so many departmental lines at such a high level.

The benchmarking project mostly disappeared from Chatsworth's radar screen at this point. At executive staff meetings he received very brief status reports, but since the other members of the executive group were on the Hess-Strickland steering committee and didn't need briefing, he did not press for more information. Instead he allowed his other responsibilities to occupy his attention. Among other things, he was in the process of educating his Board of Trustees about the current efforts to understand and address operational problems.

In fact, the benchmarking project went forward in a very conventional way. Ms. Strickland had previous benchmarking experience and soon established her role as team leader. The team was trained briefly by the person borrowed from the big hospital, who also facilitated the first few meetings. After she left, the team functioned smoothly, interacting regularly with the steering committee. At one point the CEO had to OK their team charter. He scrutinized it carefully, and when he saw that it was consistent with the agreements at the big meeting of June 18, he was satisfied and signed it. At another point a site visit was requested, which also involved a Chatsworth approval, but he was assured by Hess that the money would be well spent, so he raised no objections.

Then one day Duane Hess asked if he and Susan Strickland could meet with Chatsworth to go over a draft of the benchmarking team's recommendations. Indeed they could. How about in half an hour?

When Ms. Strickland entered the room, the CEO sensed that she was loaded for bear, so he simply welcomed her, sat everyone down, and let her go. In a matter of minutes she described the process the benchmarking team had used, who their partners had been, what questions had been asked and answered, and how the team had arrived at its recommendations. She was at pains to acknowledge the superb support she had received from the steering committee, and that they all endorsed the recommendations. She then handed Chatsworth a single piece of paper with a summary of the team's most important findings (Figure 2).

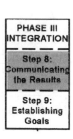

**Figure 2. Key findings.**

1. Claims processing is the weakest part of the Cranbrook Health Systems operation. Time to process, total labor hours/claim, and number of errors and omissions are 25% to 100% higher (depending upon claim category) than for the benchmarking partners.

2. Timeliness of information for effective collaboration in chemical dependency, substance abuse, and behavioral health problems is seriously deficient by comparison with benchmarking partners as measured by use of nonpanel providers. Costs of treatment in these areas is 10% to 60% higher, again depending on category of illness, for Cranbrook than for any of the benchmarking partners.

3. Case management of high-risk populations is seriously deficient, as measured by high morbidity rates, low provider continuity, poor patient education, and excess testing costs.

He read it through, and when he looked up from his reading, she handed him a second piece of paper (Figure 3) with the draft recommendations, glancing at her boss to gauge how he thought things were going. He simply smiled and nodded his head.

**Figure 3. Recommendations.**

(SUMMARY)

1. Conduct full-scale reviews of all of the major work processes of CHS. Objective: identification of opportunities for elimination of errors, delays, and duplication of effort via networked access to data. (For example: investigate potential for cost improvement if claims management is redesigned to assign to each operator all responsibility for contact with a specific set of providers.)

2. Do comprehensive redesign of claims processing and medical management based on review findings. Implement the redesigns as soon as possible.

3. Prepare a system requirements document meeting the following overall guidelines:

   • All customer-contact and provider-contact employees to have work-stations networked to each other and to the data warehouse.

   • Compatibility with St. Mark's system ensured. (The large tertiary-care hospital — the only one in the area with an up-to-date networked system.)

   • Direct access to the Cranbrook intra-net enabled for all categories of provider.

   • Requirements document to have detailed input from all work process teams, and review in draft prior to release in final form for vendor quotes. Special attention to the needs of claims processing and medical management work teams.

4. Invite vendors X, Y, and Z to prepare quotes for the Cranbrook Health Systems intra-net. (All three have full system integration capability, with strong user-support reputations.) Vendors instructed to assume initial implementation in claims processing and medical management, with flexibility maintained regarding screen detail, data flow, etc., to accommodate later extension to other major work processes after their redesign.

5. Conduct a detailed cost/benefit (and legal aspects) analysis of putting networked work-stations in all categories of provider establishment.

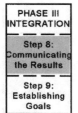

PHASE III
INTEGRATION

Step 8:
Communicating
the Results

Step 9:
Establishing
Goals

In their draft form, the recommendations were listed in chronological order. They did not refer directly to the criteria that Chatsworth and Hess had used to sort through the work process priorities, but were clearly consistent with them. (Joe Chatsworth later recalled that the benchmarking team charter's list of Requirements for Success had, however, been driven by these criteria.)

While the CEO studied the list, Susan fell silent and waited for his reaction, which was not long in coming.

"Susan, this review you start off with is clearly a *major* event. How would you propose that we structure it?" queried Mr. Chatsworth.

Thus began an in-depth discussion of the meaning and implications of the recommended actions. Joe Chatsworth was a hands-on executive and he knew his operation inside and out. Now he was led to understand where and how modern methods could increase the cost-effectiveness and quality of Cranbrook Health System's performance. However, some major changes in the work flow would be required in order to realize these benefits. The recommendations focused on these proposed actions, and so did the discussion.

The thing that finally sold Chatsworth was the common sense of it all (Susan was highly skilled at showing the conceptual simplicity underlying the complicated technical details of her specialty), plus the calm assurance with which Duane reaffirmed the full support the rest of the executive staff were giving to Susan's proposals. To make a long story short, he bought the whole package, although he noticed that there had not been much mention of how long all these recommended actions would take.

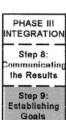

PHASE III
INTEGRATION

Step 8:
Communicating
the Results

Step 9:
Establishing
Goals

When Chatsworth finally sat back, Duane Hess spoke up, saying:

> *Joe, I know what you want to ask next: "What do I have to do to get this thing moving, and when do we start?" I'd like Susan to stay and hear what I'm about to propose. I think this woman has done an outstanding job of analyzing our organization and its needs for data processing systems. I also think that she has to be heavily involved in developing the details of the implementa-*

*tion plan and in the actual implementation. She has already been talking to potential equipment and software vendors so as to move things along more swiftly. But I think this changeover is too big and crucial to our survival to dump it all on one relatively new employee. So I'd like to suggest that we keep the steering committee going at least until we are past the initial roll-out of the new systems. With your approval, I would like to continue as a member of the committee, but shift the chairmanship to either Abbie or Doug. They have the most at stake in this transition, and I think this change in roles may be just the right move at this time.*

Chatsworth understood exactly what Hess was getting at with his proposed role changes. Abbie Aylesworth, Vice President for Customer Service Operations, and Doug Dempsey, VP Insurance Operations; were old-timers at Cranbrook and were having the most trouble coming to terms with the upheavals underway at the HMO. (In fact, both of them had come separately to him to express their concerns in private.) Joe shot his second in command a quick glance and said, "Fine. Go talk to both Abbie and Doug. Whatever you decide is all right with me. I think I'd go with Doug, if it were my choice to make. Is all this OK with you, Susan?"

Susan nodded her head and smiled. She then volunteered that the CEO would want to see the detailed implementation plan, with a milepost schedule, the detailed financials, and the manpower requirements. She also said that she assumed he would want to set the operations reviews in motion (he would), and she would present him with a detailed plan prior to the kick-off. Chatsworth agreed.

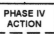

**PHASE IV ACTION**

Step 10: Developing Action Plans

Step 11: Implementing the Plan/ Monitoring Results

Step 12: Revisiting the Subject

# EPILOGUE

About six weeks after the conclusion of the benchmarking project, an evening party was given honoring its participants. The party had been suggested by Susan Strickland, but was enthusiastically supported by Joe Chatsworth. The operations reviews were going well, and his old optimism was returning by the day. At the party Chatsworth caught Susan alone for a moment and said, "How's it going with the steering committee now that Abbie is chairing it? I heard a while ago that she had some concerns about all the changes going on in the computer area."

"You heard correctly, sir," replied Susan. "But I get the feeling that she is determined to see that the steering committee does its job as well as possible, and is really digging into the details with me. I find her a tremendous help now, sort of a co-owner of the whole project."

"Sounds like the Abbie I know," was Chatsworth's comment as he drifted off to join the group around the piano.

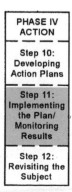

| PHASE IV ACTION |
| --- |
| Step 10: Developing Action Plans |
| Step 11: Implementing the Plan/ Monitoring Results |
| Step 12: Revisiting the Subject |

# Chapter 8

# Variations on a Theme: St. Luke's Hospital Information System Changeover

## Workforce Perspective

*Included in the workforce are all the employees of the institution not on the benchmarking team but whose work environment is affected by the actions resulting from the findings and recommendations of a benchmarking project. A few of these people may be "guest experts" called in by the benchmarking team to offer their advice in areas of special importance.*

This case study is a set of vignettes about the different experiences of several working-level employees when major changes were made in their work environment. Our story concerns what happened in a midsized community hospital when a new, integrated computerized information system was installed. We will focus on the view from the trenches in several departments during roll-out of the new system.

This case study is different from the preceding three in that it begins in Phase IV, after most of the benchmarking work has been done, and concentrates on corrective actions required during the roll-out. In the epilogue we explain how some of the difficulties encountered might have been prevented by doing things differently during benchmarking.

Things to watch for in this case study are:

> How a representative of the benchmarking team deals with a problem during implementation of the action plan (Bob's story).
>
> How a gap in the benchmarking study impacts an employee trapped in the wrong assignment because of the omission (Carol's story).
>
> How an employee behaves when he takes ownership of his part of the plan (Ralph's story).
>
> What happens when an employee who will be affected is not informed about the coming changes (Ted's story).
>
> How good communications can mitigate the effect of the inevitable glitches in the plan (Alice's story).
>
> How to identify *lessons-learned* about the benchmarking process during plan implementation.

## THE SITUATION

Saint Luke's Hospital has been using an assortment of stand-alone computer-based information systems for about 20 years. The first of these was installed in finance to handle billing. Computer use spread, slowly at first, to the laboratory, the ER, Discharge Planning, Radiology, and other areas. There have also been attempts to use computers more extensively in the bedside aspect of clinical work, but with indifferent success.

There was no coordinated planning for any of this spread of computer use, so individual department installations have different hardware, operating systems, and applications software. Communications among these systems was impossible in some cases, and difficult and frustrating where possible. Also, some of the applications software was "homemade," i.e., programmed by local people and tailored for the specific needs of a particular group. Maintenance of this software had proven to be a major headache, particularly when the user group wished to upgrade hardware and software environments. Errors and lost data had emerged as serious problems, accompanied by growing concern about ability to meet FDA and other regulatory requirements.

At the same time, and of equal importance, the managed-care revolution had made it a matter of survival for a hospital to build and maintain a complete and accurate database, both for billing purposes and for evaluating risks under capitation.

This combination of growing needs and a growing inability to perform reached crisis proportions about a year and a half ago. After intensive debate in upper management, the hospital decided to make a clean sweep — to get rid of the old piecemeal approach and put in a new integrated system. To that end, a complete study was made that involved two benchmarking projects. The goal of the first project was to find the best combination of hardware, software, and vendor for the new system. The other had the goal of determining the best process for implementing the new system. These two efforts went on roughly in parallel. The study as a whole was managed by a steering committee reporting to the COO.

Things went quite smoothly in both of the benchmarking projects. Although not required to do so by the steering committee, the two project leaders maintained informal contact with each other from time to time. They even arranged for some overlap in the choice of benchmarking partners, but there was no organized effort to integrate the two efforts more fully.

The hardware/software benchmarking project began on September 1 and concluded with vendor selection in July of the next year. System customization of a fairly routine sort took until the first of November. Installation of new hardware plus new or upgraded operating systems and applications software took place throughout the fourth quarter.

The implementation process benchmarking project began six months after the equipment selection project, on March 1, and was finished by September 1, with recommendations accepted one month later on the first of October. Roll-out to the user community began with the initial training class in the middle of the following January, right after completion of installation of the new hardware and software. During the benchmarking projects, short occasional articles appeared in the *St. Luke's News* with information on how the benchmarking work was being done and its status at the time.

## BOB'S STORY

One of the most important findings of the implementation process benchmarking team was that a major change in the information system should be piloted in one area before rolling it out to the entire user population. Also, to get the process off on the right foot in the eyes of the workforce, the pilot group should be carefully selected to have a high probability for an easy transition. It was therefore recommended by the benchmarking team that the plan should consider bringing the pharmacy into the new system first, because the pharmacy was already up on a similar platform that came from the same vendor chosen for the whole program. It was felt that the transition would be easier for the users from the point of view of familiarity of appearance of screens, keyboard conventions, commands, etc. It was also recommended that the people involved (i.e., the pharmacy) should participate in the planning.

Bob is assistant day-shift supervisor in the pharmacy, and a bit of a computer maven on his own time. When he was asked to attend a planning meeting as a "guest expert" and was told the purpose of the meeting, he was delighted. As a person with con-

PHASE IV
ACTION

Step 10:
Developing
Action Plans

Step 11:
Implementing
the Plan/
Monitoring
Results

Step 12:
Revisiting the
Subject

siderable computer literacy, he understood the likelihood of unforeseen problems. He worked diligently with the benchmarking team, and the plan he helped to develop included strong Information Systems Department support to his group. After discussing it with the head of the pharmacy, Bob concurred to the planned pilot activity and entered the trial period positively.

Things did not go well from the very beginning. Bob was frequently on the telephone with Carol, the support person from the Information Systems (IS) department. But after a few days it became clear that she was out of her depth. This came as a considerable surprise to Bob, who had identified Carol as a very strong computer type based on help she had given him with a home project involving some tricky uses of a spreadsheet program. In fact, she was considered so strong that when the details of the pilot project were being hammered out, Bob had agreed to the idea that backup support from the system vendor's help desk could be handled via an 800 number. But that arrangement had assumed only an occasional call. In the present problem-plagued situation, that was not enough. (The technical problems, which involved completely cleaning out the old operating system files on each PC so that the PC wouldn't hang under some conditions, are not our concern here, but *how they were handled* is important. This case study is about impact on the workforce.)

After a total of 10 days of frequent random PC hangs, Bob cautiously asked Carol if it might not be time to get outside help. Carol agreed, and so they called Sam Adams, the Implementation Process Benchmarking Team's designated contact person.

Sam had been chosen for his role as liaison to the workforce during implementation for several reasons. Chief among these was that he was well-known, liked, and respected by people in all of the various subpopulations in the hospital. He was patient but got things done, and almost always without ruffling anyone's feathers. When Sam learned of the problems in the pharmacy, he immediately went into action with a few well-placed phone calls. The next morning a person from the vendor's trouble-shooting squad was on the premises, and by nightfall everything was fixed.

| PHASE IV ACTION |
|---|
| Step 10: Developing Action Plans |
| Step 11: Implementing the Plan/ Monitoring Results |
| Step 12: Revisiting the Subject |

Before he left, the vendor representative remarked to Sam that, whereas the problems of the pharmacy PCs were unique to their operation, he had also found some other difficulties that would involve most of the other departments as well, and he would arrange for some comprehensive fixes when he got back to the ranch. As they shook hands, they agreed that once again the pilot approach had proven its value.

## CAROL'S STORY

Carol is the Help Desk support employee who worked with Bob on the pharmacy pilot project. As can be imagined, she did not feel good about what happened with the PCs in the pharmacy, and tended to blame herself.

The fact of the matter is that she was not given adequate preparation for her assignment — nobody thought to ask how deep her knowledge of computer systems was. It turned out that she is a whiz at using various applications that she knows well — all the commands and nifty shortcuts, etc., in her favorite spreadsheet program, for example — but she had no background in diagnosis of more subtle system-related problems.

The day after the vendor trouble-shooter's visit, Carol was talking to Sam Adams, the benchmarking team member supporting roll-out, and expressed her embarrassment about her failure. Adams responded by saying that it was not her fault, and that he planned to make it a line item in the **Lessons-Learned Report** the hospital's executive committee had asked the benchmarking team to prepare.

Adams explained to Carol that he believed the difficulty had its roots in the benchmarking questionnaire: the team had not done a sufficiently thorough job of probing its benchmarking partners about the necessary qualifications for the lead project help support person and related best practice regarding vendor backup. He went so far as to apologize to Carol on behalf of the benchmarking team for having set her up for trouble. Upon learning that nobody was blaming her because she didn't have enough depth, Carol relaxed. She accepted the apology graciously and in turn

| PHASE IV ACTION |
| :---: |
| Step 10: Developing Action Plans |
| Step 11: Implementing the Plan/ Monitoring Results |
| Step 12: Revisiting the Subject |

thanked Sam for providing such quick and effective support when it was sorely needed.

## RALPH'S STORY

Ralph is in billing. Like Bob, he also was brought into the implementation process benchmarking project as a guest expert during preparation of the recommended actions. The subject was: who should be trained first. The benchmarking team had learned that during startup there is a more or less difficult transition period when both the old system and the new system may be in use simultaneously in some work areas. The length of the transition period is dependent upon detailed work process technical considerations, and cannot be predicted accurately.

However, three of the benchmarking partners had said that in the billing function it is better initially to be able to *receive* data from an integrated database (versus *send* data to it). Thus, as the individual departments such as pharmacy, laboratory, etc., successively come on-line with the new system, the people in billing gain experience with a volume of traffic on the new system that starts small and grows. (Other advantages were discovered as well, which need not concern us here.) The only apparent disadvantage seemed to be that the billing people might be trained before they had much opportunity for hands-on experience using the new system under real-life conditions and with real data.

Ralph was brought in to share his thoughts about the proposed training schedule. He quickly saw that he would have the biggest single challenge in the roll-out plan: to initiate use of the new system in his own department and work with IS and the other departments as they learned how to get their data into the database. However, he agreed that the tradeoff was a good one. Because he was in on the planning and knew that the problems were addressed carefully, he was upbeat about the whole thing.

This plan for departmental interaction with billing during roll-out was explained to everyone in an article in *The St. Luke's News*, which pointed out that the payoff would be in the fact that the

| PHASE IV ACTION |
| --- |
| Step 10: Developing Action Plans |
| Step 11: Implementing the Plan/ Monitoring Results |
| Step 12: Revisiting the Subject |

changeover could be made with a minimum of doubling-up of database usage. The problem of keeping the billing department people's training fresh without much practice until the other parts of the user population come on line was openly acknowledged, but the tradeoff was explained and made sense to everyone. Bob was also credited in the *News* article for his part in the planning, particularly for pointing out some important details about the approach adopted, which flattered him no little.

Things got off to a good start — the training under Penelope, an excellent trainer, was done with people from billing and from the pharmacy department, because they were to be the pilot group for data input. Carol, the lead person on the help desk, was also present, and showed clearly that she had the screens and commands down cold.

There was a longer wait than anticipated for billing data to come into the new system from the pharmacy. There just wasn't much action. Ralph learned from Bob that there were startup problems, so he was patient.

After about two weeks, Sam Adams, the benchmarking project contact man, appeared and acknowledged that things had been pretty quiet, but that they would get up to speed very shortly. He sketched the difficulties the pharmacy had encountered and asked if Ralph thought some refresher training might be in order. Ralph checked with his colleagues and found that no one felt such a need. So he called Adams, thanked him for the follow-up and inquiry, but declined his offer. Clean input from the pharmacy began coming the next day.

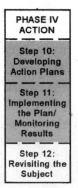

As the other departments came on-line, some links between databases were not made very well and had to be reworked to an extent. Some involved billing directly, and some did not (radiography to orthopedic floor, discharge planning to social services, internal medicine to laboratory, lab to surgery). This produced extra complications in the roll-out, and the scheduled completion of full implementation was delayed accordingly.

Since billing was involved eventually in almost everything associated with the database, Ralph was frequently in demand to offer his increasingly knowledgeable advice to medical records and other groups on how to proceed with the migration from the old system to the new one. Although he was not too thrilled about the amount of extra work required — well beyond what he had envisioned — he did this with unstinting cooperation.

"After all," he said, "the *St. Luke's News* says I was a key guy in the planning of this thing. How can I badmouth what we are doing?"

Ralph was also frequently in conversation with Sam Adams. Adams was the only person that Ralph felt he could gripe to, and one day he unloaded some rather caustic comments on Sam to the effect that if they had known what they would be getting into during the changeover period, the planning might have been done a lot more intelligently.

Instead of becoming defensive, Adams said that a Lessons-Learned report was being prepared, and he would be glad to listen to any constructively critical ideas. He mentioned, for example, that he planned to say that some of the problems could have been avoided if the two benchmarking projects had interacted sooner and more closely with each other. Adams's impression was that hardware/software/vendor selection is often not thought of as a benchmarking activity, despite the fact that most of the process steps are identical (albeit with significantly different subject matter and emphasis profiles). He had concluded that this might be the reason for the rather casual approach to communication between the two benchmarking teams, and thus the cause of the ensuing difficulties. As Adams put it in a coffee-cup conversation with Ralph, "*What* you roll out and *how* you do it are very closely related. We might have understood that more fully."

## TED'S STORY

Ted is a clerk in the administrative office of the outpatient clinic, which is located in an outlying building on the St. Luke's grounds. Ted was completely out of the loop. Somehow his group was not kept informed as the computer system program went along. All he

| PHASE IV ACTION |
| :---: |
| Step 10: Developing Action Plans |
| Step 11: Implementing the Plan/ Monitoring Results |
| Step 12: Revisiting the Subject |

heard was scary (and highly distorted) rumors. His lack of receptiveness to the new system was a major impediment to his own training and startup, and his attitude caused problems for other people as well.

Looked at with the objectivity of an outside observer, it is difficult to see why Ted was so balky. But if we look at it from Ted's point of view, the situation takes on a more complex character. So let's allow Ted to tell his own story:

*I wish I could say something good about our new information system. I guess it's going to be all right, after they get it working. But talk about confusion right now!*

*The first I heard about all this was about a year ago....Yeah, it was last Christmas. I remember someone came up to me at our holiday get-together and asked me if I had heard they were getting set to dump our whole collection of computer setups. Said they wanted to save money and had decided it was too expensive to keep our own programs up-to-date.*

*I couldn't believe my ears. When I thought of all the work we had gone through to get just the right setup for the OPD — and I have to admit it still isn't what I really want — I couldn't believe it when this same person (I forget who it was) said they were going to go with an e-mail program, and add other stuff "as needed." As needed?! All I could think was "How am I going to log patient records with an e-mail package?" Well, I didn't hear any more about it for a long time, so I guess I let wishful thinking take over and assumed it had died like a lot of other dopey ideas out of central administration. Silly me!*

*Then in July I heard they had picked a vendor for the new system. From what I was told, apparently someone's brother-in-law had an in with our Info Systems Department head, and they bought his program, even though it was not what we need and they were going to have to fix it with a lot of custom software. I really have trouble seeing why that is any different from the custom software we had to write to get our OPD computer to talk to the ones in the Pharmacy and elsewhere. Couldn't then, and can't now.*

**PHASE IV ACTION**

**Step 10:**
Developing Action Plans

**Step 11:**
Implementing the Plan/ Monitoring Results

**Step 12:**
Revisiting the Subject

*Anyway, I was talking on the 'Net with some guys I met through one of the Listservs, and they said I was lucky I had gotten any inkling at all that this fiasco was getting ready to happen. Usually they keep it all so secret you never know what hit you until it's all over. They also assured me that life was going to be sheer hell for the next year, at least, welcome to the club, and have a nice day.*

*The last straw came when I got a notice early last week saying I was scheduled for training next Tuesday, which was yesterday. Now I ask you. How could I go to training when I don't even dare get sick or take a day off because no one else can run my databases? It said arrangements would be made to take over for me. Terrific. For how many hours? For how many days? Who makes these "arrangements?" See what I mean about confusion?*

*So I called and talked to the gal responsible for the training about some of this. It came as a great surprise to her that I didn't know all about it. She was very nice, though: we spent about 15 minutes on the phone, and she filled me in on what has been happening over there in the other building (where I never go). She told me about these "benchmarking" teams, and the search for the best vendor and all. (She had never heard the stories about the e-mail package or someone's brother-in-law getting the computer order.) She also told me about the information meetings that have been announced on all the bulletin boards over there and in the* St. Luke's News *(which I never read), and what everyone else knew was coming in the way of a "roll-out schedule." I can see I have a lot of jargon to catch up on, if nothing else. She left me hoping that things wouldn't be so bad.*

*So anyway, yesterday we had the first training session and it was a disaster. Right off the bat, nobody had a word to say about why we were even doing all this stuff. So I spoke up and asked, "Why can't we just keep on improving what we already have?" Well, the trainer, a woman named Penelope who seems to know her stuff all right, gave me a little thumbnail sketch, but I had the impression that all she wanted to do was brush me off and get on with her training as quickly as possible.*

| PHASE IV ACTION |
| :---: |
| **Step 10:** Developing Action Plans |
| **Step 11:** Implementing the Plan/ Monitoring Results |
| **Step 12:** Revisiting the Subject |

*So then she started in on the new keyboard and what the function keys do in the new system. Right away I noticed a couple of other people in the class (I think there were 10 of us) were looking just as confused and unhappy as I was, and I just felt someone had to get this thing in perspective, so I said, "Who says we have to toss out everything we know and relearn a whole new set of keyboard commands and screens and stuff?" By now I was feeling sort of hot, if you must know.*

*Well, from then on it was all downhill. For instance, at one point I tried to explain that in the OPD we had tweaked our software so as to bypass some of the categories in the St. Luke's Standard Data Set that don't apply to pediatric outpatient cases, saving us a little data-entry time. I asked if this improvement could be grafted onto the new system. She didn't even know what I was talking about. Well, let 'em reinvent the wheel, see if I care.*

*Some of the other people in the class gave me pretty dirty looks as we walked out, and I heard one of them say that if I hadn't been so disruptive, they would have had more time to practice and ask questions. Me! Disruptive! All I was trying to do was get a little context for this thing so we could feel we knew why it was being crammed down our throats. Yesterday evening I checked with my friends on the 'Net and they all assured me this is the way they all act, so what was I expecting? As far as I'm concerned, there was no attempt to motivate us, or benefit from our experience, and it's not my fault that I learned precious little at their so-called training session. Now I guess I'll have to figure it out on my own. Wish me luck.*

| PHASE IV ACTION |
| --- |
| Step 10: Developing Action Plans |
| Step 11: Implementing the Plan/ Monitoring Results |
| Step 12: Revisiting the Subject |

## ALICE'S STORY

Alice is a floor nurse in internal medicine. She first learned about the new computer system from the rumor mill, but it was followed up within a few weeks by a short article on the front page of the *St. Luke's News.* From then on she got her information from the *News,* which carried brief but informative pieces every month or so, always prominently displayed. She also attended a briefing for her department and shift that was run by her supervisor and included a speaker representing the planning committee. The speaker's presentation included an announcement about the training schedule and process — how people would cover for each other, etc. This person was well informed and could answer most questions immediately, promising to get back with answers when she didn't have them on the spot.

Shortly after the briefing, Alice attended her first training session. It lasted about two hours, which just about coincided with Alice's attention span for this sort of thing. This training was in the basics of the interface to the system: security, keyboarding, certain generic screens, and so on. Alice liked the feature that automatically attached a tag identifying the person making an entry.

The class was informed that further training depended on job assignment, and on people's comfort index with what they had learned so far. At the end of the session, a woman named Carol was introduced who told them her role as the support person, and gave out her telephone number. She walked them briefly through the Help menu and some of the screens, pointing out that many people found a "cheat sheet" with some of the most-needed commands to be helpful. She was very nice, and Alice remarked to one of her friends that this sort of support would sure have been welcome year before last when we had that big clinical-support computer fiasco.

In coming weeks, Alice learned that other members of the nursing staff had had similar training experiences, although in a couple of areas, people had difficulty getting permission to attend the training. She also heard that one class had to be repeated because of disruption by a guy named Ted from the OP clinic. Alice had occasion to call Carol's Help Desk number only once, and got another person, but he was very helpful, so there was no problem.

Alice and her colleagues all had trouble communicating and sharing data with Radiology, but it was explained in an e-mail note from IS that this was a system problem that was already getting attention (an estimated date for a fix was given that turned out to be about right), and not to be frustrated.

| PHASE IV ACTION |
| --- |
| Step 10: Developing Action Plans |
| Step 11: Implementing the Plan/ Monitoring Results |
| Step 12: Revisiting the Subject |

Six months later, when everything had become reasonably routine, Alice agreed with her friend that it really hadn't been all that painful.

"It sure helped to know what was coming next, so you could brace yourself," was how Alice summarized the whole experience.

# EPILOGUE

Sam Adams made the presentation of his Lessons-Learned report to his old friends on the Implementation Process benchmarking team almost exactly a year after the team's kickoff meeting. We will not attempt to reproduce the discussion, which was very detailed, and will give only some of the flavor of his language, which was very diplomatic, as usual. These are the points he made:

1. At the very beginning, as part of Step 1 (Organizing the Project), we should have gotten agreement with all concerned to keep much closer contact with the Requirements and Vendor Selection team. Exchanging meeting minutes is not enough, and not all team members should have to be burdened with reading everything in order to find out what is relevant to both teams. I think the best way to maintain communication is to have a designated contact person for each team. This person should be familiar with what is going on in the other team and think about how it will impact what our team does.

2. We did Step 2 (Identifying the Best Practitioners) right. We maintained close enough contact with the other team so that we had some overlap in benchmarking partners. This saved us from a fair amount of misery.

3. In Step 3 (Preparing to Collect Data), our questionnaire left out one whole topic — we should have been more aggressive about finding out what is involved in providing user support. Only a few questions were needed, but we didn't think to ask them, and somehow the point never got covered in our analysis or in any of our follow-up calls.

PHASE IV
ACTION

Step 10:
Developing
Action Plans

Step 11:
Implementing
the Plan/
Monitoring
Results

Step 12:
Revisiting the
Subject

As a result of that oversight, Carol Winship needlessly went through some bad moments. You may know that on behalf of the team I told her we were sorry. It just seemed like the right thing to do (murmured agreement).

4. We did a good job with all of Phase III (Integration). It was a particularly good idea to bring in Ralph Hooper to get his thoughts on the recommendations about the training schedule. Ralph was a real trouper during the whole roll-out process.

5. In Step 10 (Developing Action Plans), we also did a lot of things right. In addition to Ralph, we got Bob Jones from the pharmacy involved in the planning. We arranged for the articles in the *St. Luke's News*, and called for the departmental information meetings, the general notices on the bulletin boards, and the individual notices about the training schedule. But we missed the Outpatient Department, and I suspect there isn't anyone who hasn't heard about Ted Baxter (vigorous nods, rolled eyes, rueful grins).

I guess the biggest lesson I learned personally is that Ted's story deserves thoughtful attention. Lord knows his language was pretty vivid, and from what I've been told, his behavior in his first training class was borderline mutinous. But his reaction, while more outspoken than most, was *not* unusual. I'm convinced that plenty of people will share his feelings if they find themselves in the same circumstances, even though they may not say a word.

You know, we inadvertently caused Ted some totally unnecessary pain. And while this isn't the place to talk about it, we also left Ted's boss with a major personnel problem. She had to call on all her experience to figure out what to do with that one. Fortunately, things are back on track, I hear.

But from a benchmarking process point of view, I think the barriers to acceptance of change raised by feelings such as Ted's, even if unexpressed, are a very real element

| PHASE IV ACTION |
| --- |
| Step 10: Developing Action Plans |
| Step 11: Implementing the Plan/ Monitoring Results |
| Step 12: Revisiting the Subject |

that will *always* accompany the process. One of the major tasks of the change agents (which is what we were) is to do everything possible to avoid ever letting those feelings become aroused. And that means *communicate*. We have to make certain that implementation planning spells out a role for every level in the chain of command down to each individual affected worker. That's in addition to the over-all communication plan we did put in place for our own situation, where everybody in the workforce was involved.

6. During Step 11 (Implementing the Plan/Monitoring Results) a few occasions came up when I had to move fast. You all know about the hiccup right at the beginning when things went off the track in the pharmacy. I only want to say that I appreciate the great support that I had from all of you whenever anything of that sort occurred. I wasn't so sure there would be much to do when I agreed to be the designated clean-up guy, but now I know better.

PHASE IV
ACTION

Step 10:
Developing
Action Plans

Step 11:
Implementing
the Plan/
Monitoring
Results

Step 12:
Revisiting the
Subject

# Part III

## Special Topics

# Chapter 9

# Benchmarking and the Internet

*"Revolution always proceeds more rapidly than expected — and evolution always proceeds more slowly than expected."*
— Anonymous

*"Forecasting is always tough, particularly when it's about the future."*
— Attributed to Casey Stengel

In Chapter 1 we pointed out that it is reasonable and natural to use contacts made *via* the Internet to search for benchmarking partners. We also mentioned that it might occasionally be appropriate to conduct other parts, or even the whole project, *via* the Internet. This chapter addresses some of the details of how to do so. It is different from the rest of the book in the sense that it departs from talking only about well-established ways of doing things and includes material that is somewhat speculative. There will inevitably be surprises, but we believe that at least some of the main ways the Internet will be useful as a benchmarking tool are already apparent.

Our basic assumption is that, with few exceptions, the changes in our ability to communicate brought about by the Internet are not going to change the fundamentals of good communications: before people will be willing to join in a benchmarking project, they will still have to have mutual interests, become acquainted, develop mutual trust, and agree on how to interact. No amount of electronic magic will change those basic requirements.

The chapter is divided into two parts. In the first part we will discuss from a benchmarking perspective some of the functional capabilities of the Internet and how they may change over time, speculating briefly on how these expanding capabilities might be useful in benchmarking-type activities. We will not dwell on specific software, hardware, service providers, or corporations, nor list specific websites — these things come and go too fast for such listings to retain reliable usefulness.

The second part will offer specific step-by-step suggestions about how the Internet might be used in a situation where the reader wishes to do part or all of the benchmarking project on the Internet.

The bibliography at the end of the book lists articles on the history and sociology of the Internet and on various practical matters related to use of the 'Net as a benchmarking tool.

## THE INTERNET AND BENCHMARKING: GENERAL

For benchmarking purposes, the following current or near-term functional capabilities of the Internet appear to be the most relevant:

| | |
|---|---|
| E-mail | Chat-room |
| Library | Document-sharing |
| Discussion Group/News Group | Voice communication |
| | Conference |

### E-MAIL

E-Mail is an excellent example of our basic assumption: big differences in degree — more, faster, more convenient — but no real differences in *kind*. E-mail is like ordinary mail. It has the advantages of ordinary mail (privacy, etc.), and suffers from the disadvantages as well (junk-mail, etc.). However, the increase in convenience, e.g., the ease of sending copies to many other people via distribution lists, and the ease of organizing one's mail for later follow-up and reference, will almost surely affect how e-mail is used in benchmarking, and deserves brief discussion.

The sheer volume of e-mail rattling around the Internet, both wanted and unwanted, has stimulated the development of powerful and ingenious software tools capable of dealing with this flood. These can be used to enrich one's benchmarking correspondence without fear of being drowned in it. For example, if you are following up a detailed fine point of some work process with several benchmarking partners at once, the automatic "threading" capability of most e-mail management programs permits one to keep track of the thread (hence the term) of the conversation, and whose contribution is whose. Similarly, the ability to create a large distribution list, and very easily send messages to everyone on it, removes an important practical barrier to seeking input from a much larger group of people. In this instance, more is better, up to a point.

## THE WORLD WIDE WEB AS A LIBRARY

The Internet is an already magnificent library. Consider the fact that in the old days, accessioning and cataloguing were labor-intensive processes performed in every library, requiring days or even weeks. The analogous functions on the Internet are now done on a daily — sometimes an hourly — basis, making the latest information immediately available in a fairly well-organized way. Over the World Wide Web the user can search the Internet "card catalogue" not only by title, author, and subject key words, but the immensely powerful search engines or "web-crawlers" even enable you to search according to collections of Boolean logic-related words of the document's text.

For example, in the preparation of the stroke case study in this book, the authors used a well-known search service to investigate information about the treatment of ischemic stroke. Searching the years 1995 and 1996, we found 4,000 citations for documents containing the words **stroke** AND **rehabilitation**, 300 citations for documents with **stroke rehabilitation**, and three for documents with **stroke rehabilitation** AND **tPA**. (AND is the Boolean "and": "x AND y" means that both x and y must be present for a hit.) On the other hand, taking a slightly different tack, we made 700 hits using **tissue plasminogen activator**, 195 using **tissue plasminogen activator** AND **stroke**, and 37 using **tissue plasminogen activator** AND **stroke** AND **clinical trials**. The point of this example is that library work hasn't changed all that much in terms of its call for imagination and persistence on the part of the user, but it has changed enormously in terms of the reward for these virtues — the search cited above took little more time to carry out than the time required here to describe what we did.

Of course, there are disadvantages as well. For one thing, there is no friendly, competent, and enormously helpful reference librarian at your elbow. You're on your own (unless you are lucky enough to get a reference librarian to do your searching for you). For another, the Web is not your local medical library. As a library it is a mix of everything you ever thought of in print, ranging from the rare books in the Library of Congress to the trivial obscenities on the men's room wall in a cheap dive.

However, it seems safe to say that any benchmarking activity that will take you to the library could also take you to the Internet, where you will often find more of what you want and find it faster if you take the time to master the available tools and resources. Moreover, you are likely to encounter valuable information not ordinarily to be found in a traditional library. For example, in the ischemic stroke search described above, several of the hits were for the CVs of people studying the use of tPA for treatment of strokes, and two were actually involved in clinical trials — possible candidates for benchmarking partners if our search had been part of a real benchmarking project.

## DISCUSSION GROUPS

By discussion groups we mean such things as the Listservs, which are e-mail based, and news groups, which are like a public bulletin board. They are both **asynchronous** — that is, the time between sending a message and receiving a reply is not fixed; it can vary from a few seconds to a week or more.

Listservs use a mail server program called Listserv, which enables a group of "subscribers" to send messages via e-mail to all subscribers to the group. There is a person designated as the "List-Owner," a moderator who serves as the gatekeeper. Mail server software automatically performs various housekeeping functions such as subscribe/unsubscribe, hold/resume, and batching for delivery. Other mail server programs such as Majordomo, Mailserv, and Mailbase have similar characteristics. Some of the mail servers support searching, but with differing levels of sophistication.

All subscribers to a mail server-supported discussion group will receive all messages posted to the server. The subscriber can then read, reply to, or ignore any of the messages posted by other subscribers. There are tens of thousands of discussion groups, commonly with subscriberships ranging into the thousands. (See the references in the bibliography for ways to find lists of discussion groups.)

News groups, of which Usenet is the dominant one, also have thousands of groups on a huge range of topics. They are similar to the mail server groups in that news server software provides groups a public forum to post information and hold discussions. The major differences between the news groups and the Listservs is that messages in news groups are posted only to the server, most news groups are not moderated (unlike the old proprietary "Bulletin Board Systems," whose population is now much diminished), and it is up to the users to query the server to find out what is new (by contrast with having all messages delivered automatically to their e-mail boxes). To make a query, interested parties use news reader software that is generally included with standard Web browsers. There is no need for the user to subscribe to a news group in order to "peek" or "lurk" around a particular news group. However, if users *do* choose to subscribe, then each time they launch the news reader application, they will be notified of new or unread messages that are still on the server for that group. News reader software also automatically provides some organization to a discussion group's messages, since related postings are presented in a hierarchical display — a discussion "thread."

Because of the asynchronous and public character of mail server and news server groups, the dynamics of these groups is like an electronic bulletin board. That is, you post your message, and after an unpredictable time lapse, someone posts a reply. Like actual physical bulletin boards, however, they are a mixed bag. They can be as orderly and well disciplined as the one outside the Anatomy Department office in a medical school, where an eagle-eyed departmental secretary (the moderator) keeps the nonsense to a minimum, or as chaotic as the one outside the coffeehouse hangout of the undergraduates, where anything goes, and usually does. In our observation, it all depends on the moderator.

For example, one discussion group with which we are acquainted began as a bonafide meetingplace for clinicians, but was allowed to be taken over by patients and their supporters and is now used as an extended support group. Is this bad? No, but it is different from the original intent, and the clinicians have understandably moved on to a different location on the Internet. As another example, an otherwise extremely orderly and well-run Listserv went off on a tumultuous side-track over a Christmas holiday, when the List-Owner was on vacation. It came back on track as soon as she returned, with no great harm done.

It is amazing (and heartwarming) the lengths to which people with a mutual interest will go to help each other *via* discussion groups. Those familiar with Listservs will agree that it is not at all unusual for a very respectable annotated bibliography in some highly specialized technical area to be produced by a subscriber in response to a call for help from a colleague.

It is equally possible to get very impressive-looking input from prestigious e-mail addresses based on nothing but strongly held opinions. For example, if your project is tightly focused on learning about the best equipment and practices in making a blood draw, you will probably do very well using the Internet. But if your concerns extend to *who should do the draw*, be prepared for a much more diffuse set of responses.

From the benchmarking point of view, a good discussion group is like much fine gold. With it, you can seek potential benchmarking partners, obtain information about experience using specific products, processes, and vendors, get advice about complying with various government regulations and regulatory bodies, and even engage in high-quality (albeit asynchronous) dialogue on policy matters relevant to the central interests of the particular group.

The main catch is that you have to dig for what you want. As mentioned above, the search capability may be limited, and "threading" is comparatively cumbersome (but bound to improve with time) if the subscriber depends entirely on the mail-server software. A more important limitation, however, is that response to your inquiry is strictly voluntary. Thus, you may get a huge response or no responses, and have to resort to other methods. For example, an inquiry about an unpopular illness may be ignored, while one with a large following may call forth an avalanche of replies.

Also, even though there may be a large number of subscribers to a particular discussion group, only a small fraction of them may be active enough so that you feel you "know" them. Listserv subscribers are encouraged to provide a CV when they sign on to some listserv discussion groups, but this doesn't always happen. So, you may throw out a question, and get responses from people whose qualifications will be unknown to you, and follow-up inquiry becomes necessary.

## Chat Rooms (Chat Corners, etc.)

Like real rooms, chat rooms can be public or private, orderly or disorderly, comfortable/safe/rewarding, or the exact opposite. For benchmarking purposes, we can safely restrict attention to private (by invitation only) discussion sites for a specific area of subject matter, with a designated moderator (yourself or your computer expert). With this as the focus, a chat room can be thought of as the text-based equivalent of a moderated telephone conference call.

Anyone who has participated in an ordinary telephone conference call of five or more people whose voices are not easily recognized by each other understands the advantage of being able to identify each participant's contributions. The keyboarded equivalent has this advantage, of course, plus the fact that a transcript of the discussion, including previously prepared supporting documentation if you wish, is prepared automatically. Chat-rooms do have other characteristics all their own, however, which should be experienced directly (and practiced!) before you decide to use them for benchmarking. For example, it can be unnerving to the newcomer to see how quickly some participants appear to be entering their comments, not knowing that frequently used questions and remarks are being pasted in from an existing collection.

## Document-Sharing/"White Boards"

Document-sharing on the Internet is possible at more than one level. At its most elementary, a file can be pasted into, or attached to, an e-mail message for transmission to a receiver for later attention (asynchronous mode). Doing this is very easy if both sender and receiver are on the same intra-net, use the same kind of computer and have the same applications programs running. However, when the document is sent from one kind of computer platform, has to leave its local network, pass fire-walls and through the 'Net servers of a hodgepodge of service providers, and ends up at a computer with a different operating system running different applications, things are very different. Software to deal with these problems is changing rapidly, however, and one can hope that it will soon be possible to do this seemingly simple chore without worrying about running a gauntlet of protocols, compatibilities, and busy signals.

A more advanced capability is the synchronous mode, in which two people can have the same document file open on linked computers so that they can work on it simultaneously, much as if they were standing together in front of a white board. As can be imagined, the compatibility requirements here are more stringent, and, depending on the configuration of the link-up, there can be technical issues involving file update strategies and bandwidth requirements to avoid annoying screen refresh delays. We project that these also will be surmounted in time.

The real question, however, is how useful all this technically sophisticated "meetingware" will be. The answer probably lies in the stage of preparation of the document under consideration. Probably not too useful in the early stages, more so when doing final clarification and polishing. How often is it that two people wish to sit down to write a document or draw a flow-diagram from scratch *together*? Experience with so-called collaboratories is still relatively skimpy, but the indications are that creation is still a basically solitary activity; only one person at a time actually draws the line, writes the sentence or does the calculation. People seem to perform better when some suitably sized unit of work is presented for critique. This will be different from person to person and subject to subject, to be sure, but we project that the benefits of synchronous document-sharing are more likely to lie in the ease of rapid response to a piece of work already in draft, thus enabling faster iteration, but not so much in literal simultaneity at all stages.

Thus, in a benchmarking project where two partners are conferring via the Internet about a draft report involving text, figures, and perhaps spreadsheets, it may some day be very helpful for both parties to have the same page on their screens at the same time, with the ability to move back and forth simultaneously among different pages prepared with different applications programs.

## Voice Communication

The telephone system is quite a remarkable achievement, as those who are learning to duplicate its capabilities on the Internet have discovered.

The Internet equivalent of voice mail will soon be attractive in terms of affordable user hardware and software. However, because of its relatively high bit-content — much higher than text, although much lower than video or complex graphics — voice-mail will add correspondingly to the congestion on the information highway. The advent of Internet 2 (a high-speed fiberoptic digital network being established among research institutions) will do much to alleviate this congestion for users in the government and academic world.

## CONFERENCES

It is becoming increasingly practical to combine features of all of the modalities described above into a conference. The threading capability of e-mail, the synchronous, record-building capability of chat-rooms, the ability to share documents, and, increasingly, voice communications as an integral part of the package, are all now available bundled into single conferencing programs. Running them is not child's play, however, and for the foreseeable future will require, in addition to the moderator, experienced computer types for administration, particularly regarding compatibility issues and problems associated with use of the telecommunications network. Nevertheless, we project that the day of decentralized full-capability video-conferencing, with its advantages of being able to see and hear the other conferees while discussing a document, a drawing, or a piece of new equipment, is surely coming.

## PEOPLE ISSUES

The *technical* aspects of the Internet are clearly revolutionary, and have driven the spread of its use at a breathtaking pace, particularly with the arrival of the 'Net-surfing general public. The social aspects of the 'Net are not nearly so clear, however, and some of them may turn out to be more evolutionary in character. Human nature changes very slowly, and it may be that people (liveware?) issues will set the pace of change in some directions. Although it is not within the scope of this chapter to analyze human dynamics or community-building on the Internet, a couple of examples may help to illustrate what we have in mind about how human behavior could affect the direction and pace of change.

- The tendency to seek your own kind. Specialists in a field have an uncanny way of discovering each other, and for erecting barriers against intruders. The Internet will make it easier for candidates for membership in these informal clubs to **search** for them. It may not be so easy to **find** them, however and to learn of their existence and whereabouts in cyberspace. Web pages come and go, and the easiest thing in the world is to form a small subset of a group that has become too large, and set up a new address where a more narrowly specified interest group can "meet" to exchange ideas and information. Call it the "Robin Hood effect" if you will: in a big dense forest, it is easy to achieve privacy. This could work either for or against you in the benchmarking context.

- The larger the total population to choose from, the easier it will be to find enough people to keep your need for professional company satisfied with a narrower and narrower definition of whom you wish to talk to. Think of it as a kind of "inverse tragedy of the commons"— nobody needs to go to the village commons for somebody to talk to anymore. One bad effect of this withering of the sense of community would be the drying up of cross-fertilization of ideas from one specialty to another. Some believe this could already be happening to a number of specialties, and refer to it as a "balkanization effect" (Van Alstyne and Brynjolfsson 1996, 1479). Benchmarking, on the other hand, usually requires a multidisciplinary mind-set, and may not appeal to tightly focused specialists who are only interested in communicating with their specialist colleagues.

## SUMMARY APPRAISAL

The Internet seems to be good at providing some things that can be useful in benchmarking:

a. Information and advice about specific work processes and their details.

b. Information about a person's interests and qualifications.

c. Information and advice about experience with specific products or vendors.

d. Information and advice about regulatory requirements at federal, state, and local levels.

To this list of potentially helpful characteristics of the Internet must be added the caveats we have already mentioned plus some others that we will take up in context in the next section on the detailed use of the Internet in benchmarking.

# BENCHMARKING VIA THE INTERNET

## GENERAL

There are obvious incentives for wanting to do a benchmarking project on the Internet: you may expect to save time or money, or you believe you will get better results, or you think the project might be easier to do, or some combination of these. These are reasonable things to hope for. Clearly if you can take full advantage of the power of the 'Net you will significantly broaden the base of potential benchmarking partners, you can get answers to your questions more quickly, and you may be able to avoid the cost of site visit travel.

Fortunately, there are many situations where these benefits can indeed be captured. It frequently happens that a need is not big enough to warrant a full-blown benchmarking project, but is too big or too urgent to be ignored. For example, if the need is focused on one or a few of the work processes and outputs of a single unit or department, and you are in a hurry, the Internet route may be entirely satisfactory. An amazing amount of very helpful information is available, sometimes enough to produce all the benefits of a formal project, but without the concomitant expenditures of time and money.

However, whether this actually leads to better results or truly makes the project less costly overall depends on avoiding some potential pitfalls.

*Results.* The results of a benchmarking project are measured by the successful adoption or adaptation of best practices from outside the organization. You may be very successful in *finding* these best practices *via* the Internet, but discover that getting them *accepted* in your own institution is hampered by lingering wariness of their source in cyberspace. In many, if not most, organizations at this writing, the Internet has not yet achieved the wide acceptance as a source of solid information and sound counsel that its best offerings deserve. Particularly in the higher reaches of management, there is often a lack of familiarity with the Internet, which reduces the influence of information and ideas obtained from it. Be sure that the people with decision authority to implement the recommendations based on your findings are comfortable with their source. If the subject is sufficiently restricted in scope so that only a few like-minded 'Net fans are needed to take advantage of what you have learned, quick acceptance of input from the 'Net should be expected. Otherwise, be prepared for more lengthy discussions.

*Project cost.* In thinking about the cost of an Internet benchmarking project, it is important to assess the availability of computer expertise a resource that may be scarce, and therefore relatively costly, in your institution. You will want all benchmarking team members to be comfortable with e-mail and word processing, and at least one person should be familiar with a flow-charting program. But if you are planning to do a site visit *via* the Internet, you may need help from someone with broader knowledge of 'Netware. Such experts may be in very short supply, which will inevitably drive up the cost in either time or money. Also, there may be security concerns that require encryption software, driving up the cost of communication.

It may turn out that your electronic site visit does not work out well and a conventional visit is needed, resulting in lost time. This is most likely to happen when you discover that it is more important than you had thought to actually *see* what the partnering organization is doing and/or the environment in which they are doing it. As a simple example, the width of corridors, their lighting, traffic levels, and the amount of clutter tolerated can impact patient transport times. If your team has representatives on the spot, it is less likely that misconceptions will occur. If you are trying to stitch together the best suggestions from several Internet participants in a study, you must take care that details of this sort are not lost without anyone realizing it.

Or it may happen that the Internet approach to conferencing just doesn't go well because your conference is a first attempt at using this tool, also leading to need for a conventional visit. We will talk later about a way around this latter danger, but it involves practice, which also adds to the cost.

So far we have been talking about how *you* will use the Internet in benchmarking. However, anyone in your organization is free to use the Internet, and how they use it can have a dark side as well.

A frequent problem with benchmarking projects is that the scope of the required changes in the work processes of various groups is underestimated. Such situations are always touchy, but the Internet tends to increase their volatility. The reason is that there are all sorts of interest groups on the 'Net who develop an in-group way of thinking about their particular interest. This can lead specialists in your organization to seek advice and support from colleagues in their specialty when they feel threatened by a proposed change in what they are doing. If the proposed change is presented to Internet buddies in an incomplete or distorted form, the advice or support they get may strengthen any natural inclination to dig in their heels and resist the proposed changes. For example, in the Information System Upgrade case study in Chapter 8, Ted, the data clerk, has his worst fears amplified by friends on the Internet and his behavior becomes a real problem.

## STEP-BY-STEP

Under appropriate circumstances as discussed above, all the activities in Phases I and II of the benchmarking process — from Selecting the Subject to Updating the Findings and Recommendations — can be carried out in whole or in part using the Internet as a tool. Phases III and IV, on the other hand, are both done in-house, so potential Internet involvement will be minimal.

The following are some suggested modifications to the individual steps in the benchmarking process to accommodate partial or full use of the Internet.

### Phase I: Planning

Step 1: Organizing the project. Obviously, the Internet can help significantly to broaden everyone's awareness of the outside world. In management debates about strategic priorities, more and more accurate awareness is crucial to sound judgments about priorities. However, in this context the Internet is only one more source of information; it is not a tool for priority-setting.

Picking the team personnel, however, will be more strongly affected by an intent to use the Internet. Obviously you will want a leader who is sufficiently familiar with the Internet to be able to orchestrate the activities and schedule knowledgeably. Perhaps less obvious is the need for a sponsor who is acquainted with the Internet, and strongly supportive of its use for benchmarking.

You will also need at least one team member with computer expertise more advanced than only as a user of e-mail. It probably is not necessary for all team members to be adept in use of the Internet, but everyone who anticipates being involved in Internet conferences at the later stages of the project must be comfortable with use of the applications programs you intend to use. This should be kept in mind during team selection and training, if any.

Step 2: Identifying the best practitioners. *Self-initiated approach*. If you are already familiar with the World Wide Web in its capacity as a library, you can use one of the existing search engines to canvass your chosen subject very efficiently. If you are not familiar with the Internet, ask your reference librarian or someone who can fill that function to look for sites where you can go to make inquiries. Interested individuals in discussion groups such as the listervs may respond to a posted inquiry. But remember that your inquiry is now viewable by a large audience.

Another approach is to post an e-mail message to a list of existing contacts or people whom you locate via address lists from a professional society meeting or industry forum such as the meetings of the Institute for Healthcare Improvement. This approach has the advantage that the messages can be tailored to the individual or subpopulation you are addressing, and, of course, they are much more private.

*Group approach*. If you are thinking of joining in a group benchmarking project, for example with the American Academy of Pediatrics or the College of American Pathologists, group requirements will determine how you proceed regarding protocols, operating environment (Mac, DOS, or Unix), applications programs, etc.

Whichever approach is taken, however, don't do your thinking on the Internet. Positioning the project should be done ahead of time — your benchmarking project scope and the aggressiveness of your improvement goals should be reflected in the wording of the messages you send out. The spoken word, the sped arrow, and the sent Internet message cannot be recalled.

Step 3: Preparing to Collect Data. If you are doing your project on the Internet, try to have everything possible in digital form and thus ready for transmission under program control. Fortunately, there are many excellent applications program tools available for quality-oriented projects. For example, you may choose to begin flowcharting the process you wish to improve on a blackboard, but get it into digital form as soon as possible using flowcharting software.

If you are doing a project in which existing databases will be involved, you will want to conform to the reporting standards established for them.

When recruiting benchmarking partners (as distinguished from seeking candidates, covered above in Step 2), placing total reliance on the Internet may not be wise. Try to feel out which would be the better approach — more e-mail or a timely telephone call — and act accordingly. People differ widely in their reactions on this score.

## Phase II: Data Collection and Analysis

Step 4: Administering the questionnaire. The preferred method of administering the questionnaire always is by mail, and e-mail has some important advantages (see Chapter 2). There are two caveats, however:

1. Be sure that the formatting of the questionnaire, which is an important aspect of its user-friendliness, is preserved in transmission. This may require some experimentation. Also, given the current state of the art in e-mail technology, don't assume that just because the questionnaire went to one recipient without a hitch, it will go the same way to all of them. Follow up each transmission to see that it came through unmutilated.

2. Discuss with your respondents what they plan to do with the questionnaire upon receipt. If their first move will be to reroute individual sections to specific people for response by e-mail, they may appreciate an offer to send the sections directly to these people. (Of course, if the contact's first move will be to print out the questionnaire before responding *by hand* you might well ask whether this is a good choice of benchmarking partner for the Internet approach.)

Step 5: Analyzing the data. One of the chief benefits of sending the questionnaire by e-mail and receiving it the same way is that data compilation is easier (see Chapter 2). Take advantage of this opportunity by making sure during the screening process that this approach is acceptable to potential benchmarking partners.

Clarifying follow-up with respondents is also easier by e-mail, and so is distribution of the clarified and annotated compilation of the results to other benchmarking team members. Be sure, however, that any clerical work done by a nonteam member is reviewed before distribution.

Step 6: Identifying best practices. Recall from Chapter 2 that there is one very important meeting of the benchmarking team that has three related objectives: to understand how best practices work, to identify the greatest opportunities for improvement, and to begin preparing conclusions and recommendations for action. You should consider conducting this meeting electronically, using document-sharing or even conferencing software programs if you foresee the possibility of an electronic site visit. This may seem a little artificial, but we believe it is justified as practice or a *rehearsal* for similar meetings that you plan to conduct *via* the Internet with benchmarking partners at remote locations. If you do choose to follow this approach, be sure it is facilitated by someone skilled in the use of the software involved, and that this person is alert to opportunities to make the process go more smoothly.

Step 7: Doing site visits (on the Internet). One of the main reasons for benchmarking *via* the Internet is to avoid site visits. You will have ascertained your benchmarking partners' ability and willingness to participate in Internet-based meetings during the screening process. Now prepare your team well for them, and urge your partners to do the same. It is not overkill to divide your team into two subgroups and conduct a mock meeting for practice. Remember, it would take a lot longer to climb on an airplane and travel 1,000 miles for a face-to-face session!

All other preparation should be done just as if an actual visit were in the offing: assignment of roles, development of detailed lists of in-depth probes, etc.

### Phase III: Integration, Phase IV: Action

The last two Phases of a benchmarking project are done in-house, and there are only a few things remaining to be said about use of the Internet.

- Recalling the point made earlier about resistance to change, it is in Phases III and IV that you can expect the negative aspects of the Internet to show up. Your project is now up for widespread in-house scrutiny, and unconvinced individual professionals may resort for solace and support to like-minded Internet cronies. Do not be surprised to find messages on the intra-net in your organization that have been pulled in from distant locations to refute and/or undermine your conclusions and recommendations. It won't matter whether they are distorted, or out of context, or just plain wrong; the impact will be there, and you must be prepared to deal with them. Forewarned is forearmed.

- When approaching decision-making management to explain your project's approach, results, and recommendations, be very sensitive to the individual preferences of your audience. There is still an enormous range of personal attitudes toward computers, the Internet, and all they represent. You will have executives who pride themselves on how fast they respond to their e-mail, and you will have people like the professor (not a fictional creation) who will only use e-mail to let you know a fax is coming. Unquestionably, it will be easier to transmit material that is already on disk to key individuals electronically, but you have to ask yourself whether that is the easiest way to *communicate* with them. The object is to persuade, not dazzle.

- In Step 10, Developing Action Plans, the responsibility for detailed planning is handed off to the people who will have to implement the plan. You will be tempted to pressure them to use some of the powerful and (to you) nifty software tools you have become proficient with. Don't do it. As we have said repeatedly, your objective is to improve how the work gets done. If they show interest in using Internet-related software, by all means be there to help, but serving as a flack for the latest in shrink-wrap is not part of that picture.

# Chapter 10

# Benchmarking Healthcare Costs

*Cost plays a pivotal role in all businesses at all times. Outside healthcare, it is the one subject most likely to surface when you ask a busy executive what she spends most time thinking about. Cost and its management are involved one way or another in practically all industrial benchmarking projects. Healthcare now shares this same preoccupation with cost.*

It seems safe to say that the healthcare sector will concentrate hard on cost, its definition, measurement, control, and most especially its reduction, for the indefinite future. And it will not be an easy situation to deal with. This focus on cost has already produced deep rifts within healthcare itself and between healthcare organizations and the public. Some in the caregiving community try to fend off any attempts to manage cost in the conscientious belief that such attempts are diametrically at odds with the integrity of the care-giving function. Other interested parties are equally zealous in their belief that only through the application of business-management techniques can the *value* of healthcare — quality of service delivered at a given cost — be raised to affordable levels. Somehow these points of view must be reconciled. Mutual understanding of the facts is one of the keys to success, and here is where benchmarking can be a great help.

This chapter is devoted to the benchmarking of healthcare cost. The chapter is broken into two parts: a general discussion of cost seen from the benchmarking point of view, followed by a discussion of the application of benchmarking to one very important cost-related issue — the transition to a capitated environment. There will not be, however, any discussion of the how-to mechanics of cost accounting, which is outside the scope of this book.

# GENERAL CONSIDERATIONS

## DEFINITION OF COST

At first glance, it might seem a bit pedantic to worry about the definition of cost; at the simplest level everyone knows what cost is. For benchmarking purposes, however, we need to know *what to include* and *where to include it* in our definition of the cost of something.

### What to include

We are all aware of the problem of identifying all the costs of electric power. We know there is more to that cost than what is on our utility bill every month. We have learned, to our sorrow, that the total cost of power to society should include, for example, the cost of the acid-rain pollution produced by coal-burning power plants. But because this cost is not included in our utility bills, we don't know how big that cost is. If New York State were to clean up all the lakes in the Adirondacks, what would it cost? Nobody knows because no generally accepted estimate has ever been made.

Another familiar example comes from within healthcare: What is the cost of a JCAHO accreditation site visit? (Note that we are focusing here only on the *cost* of a familiar activity — not questioning its *benefits*.) At one 350-bed community hospital, the out-of-pocket fee to the Joint Commission for a recent survey was $38,000. But that was not the total cost of this hospital's JCAHO accreditation. The hospital also has one person on the staff who works full-time on JCAHO matters, and during the year of the visit at least two additional FTEs were involved in preparation for the visit. Assuming an average total compensation/year of $50,000 for the people involved, a conservative estimate of the cost of this accreditation is thus closer to $200,000 during the year of the site survey, and somewhat over $50,000 in the off-years. You can probably think of dozens of other examples of this sort.

## Where to include it (Allocation)

In the acid-rain example given above, not only do we not really know what the cost of clean-up would be, we also don't know *whose* cost it should be — whose utility bill it should it be added to. Nobody knows because the issue has never been decided, either legislatively or judicially.

Issues associated with allocated costs come up repeatedly in manufacturing industries. As late as the mid-80s, for example, it was not uncommon in some industries to allocate the cost of all supervisory and administrative staff, and even the cost of plant and machinery amortization (all *indirect* costs) to unit labor cost (a *direct* cost). The ludicrous result was a calculated "cost per hour" for an assembly-line worker running into the thousands of dollars.

Healthcare is not exempt from the dilemmas of allocation. For example, in a hospital's total utility bill, what fraction is allocated to the surgical suites? Very probably nobody knows because the subject has never come up. But if it did, any number of elements of the total cost would have to be considered and allocated. For instance, how should the capital cost of the emergency generators necessary to run vital services during a power outage be allocated? You may not even want to think of the cost of that generator as being part of the utility cost, preferring to think of it rather as part of the institution's insurance budget instead. It is because of considerations like this that financial analysts in industry say that you should not try to define or allocate costs until you know what you want to do with them.

Note that these kinds of allocation decisions need not be difficult in themselves. As long as it is done in a way that avoids leaving out a cost element or double-counting it, there is nothing conceptually difficult. Serious problems can arise, however, if the situation is overlaid with a cost-cutting objective, and departmental goals are set. Then the definition of cost, and whose cost, can become quite contentious. Simple matters of cost allocation can lose their logical focus and turn into highly divisive turf wars in such circumstances.

The definition and allocation of a cost can have important practical consequences for benchmarking. For example, suppose a benchmarking team is asked to seek out best practices for reducing the *direct cost* of a work process that makes heavy use of computer systems. Suppose further that the computer systems involved are considered to be an indirect cost in this organization (a common situation), allocated across the user population according to a formula that does not include the actual marginal cost of usage. If the benchmarking team does not think to explore opportunities to find more cost-effective computer support for their work process, it would hardly be surprising. Situations like this abound, and provide a strong incentive for the adoption of Activity Based Costing (ABC) an accounting formalism that enables the allocation of costs on a strict usage basis. Under Activity Based Costing, all resource usage, either money or supplies, or people's time, is assigned to specific activities and then to the products or services these activities support. A concerted effort is made to reduce — ideally eliminate — allocation of indirect cost according to some general formula unrelated to actual use.

From the benchmarking perspective, the main thing is to be sure that you have a list of all the elements you wish to include in your cost clearly in mind before you compare with your benchmarking partners, and ensure that both organizations are including the same cost elements when you compare totals. In the accreditation site visit example given above, it is obvious that Hospital A, which counts only its out-of-pocket fee, would be shocked to learn what Hospital B's accreditation visit total cost is if they don't know that Hospital B counts personnel time as well.

But it is still not enough to include people's time all lumped into one category. To get a good comparison between how you and your benchmarking partners prepare for an accreditation survey, it is far more illuminating to list how much administrative management time, how much medical staff time, etc., are expended in the survey process. Thus, you may find, for example, that you do not have a clerk assigned to JCAHO matters full-time, but that your CEO spends the equivalent of a month during the year of the survey on the survey itself and a batch of follow-up actions, while your benchmarking partner estimates three equivalent days of CEO attention, but does have two clerks assigned full-time. Useful comparison of the two organizations requires all this information.

## Cost Definition and Cost Allocation Guidelines

- Make a complete list of all the elements you intend to include in your definition of the cost of the service you are benchmarking and obtain concurrence from key stakeholders.

- Be sure that allocation of cost elements is done with agreement of the stakeholders, particularly when cost-reduction programs are involved.

# MEASUREMENT OF COST

We mentioned above that some say you should not try to define or allocate costs until you know what you want to do with them. The same applies to the **measurement of cost**. To illustrate this point, let us assume that Hospital A is considering marketing some of its laboratory services to other organizations in the area. Hospital A has decided to include some blood products in its offering, and recognizes that it may be necessary to establish satellite locations to facilitate rapid delivery. In order to set prices for the various functions they plan to offer, Hospital A people will need to know their costs for these functions. (CAVEAT: because of antitrust laws, NEVER attempt to benchmark PRICE.)

As part of its feasibility study, Hospital A decides to benchmark the cost of delivery of the blood products in the marketing plan. It now becomes necessary to break out the cost of the specific work processes used to deliver these blood products, and to understand the *real* costs, as opposed to the *allocated* costs, of the work environment (building, utilities, equipment/equipment maintenance, etc.) that must be provided for the blood bank to operate in a satellite location.

Contrast this situation with the one in the first benchmarking case study in Part II, where the blood bank at Good Samaritan hospital is benchmarking its services with the objective of improving the processes by which blood components are distributed by the blood bank. The Good Samaritan study is focused primarily on reducing errors and late delivery to the users. The main thing Good Samaritan needs to do is understand the work flow involved in providing its principal services, allocating many of its costs across the whole range of the services it provides. Thus, even though cost is involved in the Good Samaritan case, from a benchmarking perspective Hospital A, which is planning to market its services selectively, and in a different physical setting, has need for a much more detailed breakdown of the cost information.

It will probably be necessary for Hospital A to bring financial people into the benchmarking project on an active basis in order to cost out the activities in the relevant work process flow diagrams because most healthcare organizations do not measure cost this way. They do not accumulate cost data either at this level of detail, or broken down in such a way as to be useful in understanding costs for individual products.

When doing detailed cost comparisons, it is a good idea to include the *primary metrics* for each item in your list of cost elements. For example, in the accreditation site visit discussed earlier, fees to the Joint Commission would be given in *dollars* as the primary metric, while CEO time, medical staff time, etc., would be listed in *hours* or *days* as the primary metric. These can later be converted into dollars with suitable conversion factors if it is desired to have an overall total dollar figure.

## Cost Measurement Guidelines

- Measure at a level of detail consistent with the objective of the benchmarking project.

- Both line and financial staff people should participate.

- Include primary metrics (staff time in hours or days, fees in dollars, medication in dosage units. etc.)

Demanding as these actions may appear to be, there is no escape from them in a competitive world. If you can't measure your costs, how can you possibly learn how to reduce them in order to stay competitive? You might say that it doesn't matter all that much to know exactly what the details of our costs are, as long as we are actively working to reduce them. Indeed this may be so. But how can you be sure you are working on the right parts of the cost picture? A lot of wasted effort results when you give high priority to reducing a cost element that accounts for 1% of the total, while ignoring another one that makes up 20% of the total, and is capable of being significantly reduced. (See Cost Of Poor Quality.)

230

## CONTROL OF COST

Cost control in American business has become a partnership between finance and line management. The traditional record-keeping function of accounting, with periodic reporting to upper management, has evolved into a closely coupled interaction between financial analysts and the line managers at all levels to whom they are assigned as support, with almost real-time availability of financial performance information in some industries. One benefit of this change has been to enable much more rapid detection of situations that show signs of getting out of control, leading to more nuanced corrective actions that are not as disruptive to operations. When applied to the flow of materials, for example, it has led to the much-praised "just-in-time" (JIT) inventory cost control systems, where minimal stocks of supplies are maintained and replenished as needed by the vendors.

The recent increase in adoption and use of JIT for various categories of supply items in healthcare institutions is a harbinger of more to come. But it is largely the result of interaction between the finance and purchasing functions, and for the most part the actual caregiving functions still do not benefit from a finance/operations partnership. It is still all too common that at the level of first-line supervision in the clinical functions, costs are, if anything, simply recorded, not controlled.

### Reduction of cost

Cost control factors also apply to cost reduction, but to a much more critical degree. The reason is easy to see: cost control is about monitoring financial performance to see that the cost of doing things in the usual way do not get out of hand; cost reduction is about changing the cost of what we do by changing what we do or the way we do it. Past experience is a reasonably good indicator of future performance in a stable operation. But when the objective is to change all that, deeper understanding of the key operational drivers of output quality, and more detailed knowledge of the key elements that drive the cost of operations is essential. Successful cost reduction requires partnership between financial analysts and line personnel, starting with the benchmarking phase. Thus, the relatively arm's-length relationship between finance and operations, particularly clinical operations, must be changed whenever a benchmarking project has a strong cost focus. It will not do, for example, to have a benchmarking team that is addressing the cost of MRI diagnostics with only radiology department people or only finance people on the team. When the time comes to make recommendations for cost improvement goals, both are needed in order to examine the vital links between the steps we carry out in our work process and the costs associated with each of these steps.

### Cost Reduction Guideline

- Always include both functional people and financial people in any benchmarking project where cost reduction is an objective.

## COST OF POOR QUALITY (COPQ)

COPQ is a process tool for identifying areas where customer requirements are not being met and prioritizing the opportunities for improvement. It is *a very valuable estimating tool,* whose principal application is strategic — when used for seeking out and prioritizing major opportunities for cost reduction and quality improvement it can't be beat. A COPQ estimate is very useful when you want to arrive at an order of magnitude estimate of the size of a cost problem. It is most easily used for questions like:

- Are we wasting $1M a year in performing service X, or only $100K?
- Is the waste in performing service X twice as large as the waste on service Y, or only half as large?

Consistency in its application is far more important than precision, particularly when tracking progress over time.

The proper mental preparation for using COPQ might go something like the following:

- Our basic objective is to become and remain competitive.
- Satisfying our customers' requirements is the surest way to do this sustainably.
- Not meeting customer requirements, for whatever reason, is *wasteful of scarce resources.* Moreover, doing things that are for the purpose of meeting customer requirements, but *doing them ineptly* is also wasteful of scarce resources.

# DEFINITIONS

## Cost of Conformance

| | |
|---|---|
| • Cost of Prevention | Cost incurred to keep failure from happening. (Failure means having to redo or correct a service already performed.) *Example:* Repetitive verification of patient's drug allergies prior to surgery. |
| • Cost of Appraisal | Cost incurred to measure conformance to quality standards. *Example:* Accreditation site visits. |

## Cost of Nonconformance

| | |
|---|---|
| • Cost of Internal Failure | Cost of correcting a service prior to delivery to the customer. *Example:* Discard of expired blood products |
| • Cost of External Failure | Cost of correcting a service after delivery to the customer. *Example:* Unscheduled readmission after discharge. |

## COST OF POOR QUALITY IS ESSENTIALLY A MEASURE OF WASTE

The authors acknowledge Mr. C. Caldwell's contribution to this topic. In his book *Mentoring Strategic Change in Health Care,* Caldwell distinguishes *efficacy* (doing the right things) and *efficiency* (doing things right). Caldwell's basic point is that doing things that don't add value is wasteful.

There are several traps for the unwary in using the COPQ tool. Understanding them will help you to deal with them successfully.

- There can be a lot of subjectivity and ambiguity in COPQ. It is one of those terms like *art* and *beauty* that can become very complicated very quickly. As in all matters having to do with cost, it is hard to know what to include and what to leave out. But beyond that, detailed dissection of a particular activity can lead to all sorts of terminology and classification problems. For example, a JCAHO accreditation site visit is a Cost of Conformance, and spending money on ensuring conformance to requirements is generally agreed to be A Good Thing. But there can be smoothly executed site visits, with no loose ends, and other kinds of visits that require a great deal of frantic preparation, updating of records, cleanup of work areas, follow-up actions, etc. Are both kinds of site visits to be classified the same way, or does the untidy visit actually have some Cost of Nonconformance mixed into it? Other examples can be even harder to unravel.

Because of this potential for subjectivity and ambiguity, most financial people are uncomfortable with COPQ, and most accounting systems are not set up to gather COPQ data as such. Sometimes a separate tracking system for Cost of Poor Quality is set up, but there is a risk that tracking can become an objective for its own sake. This is particularly likely to happen if a COPQ bureaucracy is set up.

• It is hard to get people to admit that *their* activities are contributing to waste and lowered customer satisfaction, and territorial reflexes are easily triggered by COPQ studies. COPQ is not good, and if two or more organizations contribute in series to providing a single service with a large COPQ, then the temptation is to blame the group or person upstream/downstream from you in the work flow for your problems. ("If the lab hadn't taken so long with the biopsy, I wouldn't have kept the patient on the operating table so long."/"We can't trust floor people to get the lines inserted correctly, so we get them started before the patient leaves the recovery room — that's why we take so long.") Unfortunately, there is sometimes enough truth in such accusations that attention is drawn away from the real issues, which are usually *system problems*: problems at the interface between the interacting units. In a tightly compartmentalized organization, the temptation to blame people in other units for COPQ problems is very prevalent, but deficiencies in the system are almost always the root cause of failure to meet customer requirements in a cost-effective manner.

Due to the normal human tendency to deny and to export our problems rather than to admit and to solve them, it is of the utmost importance to remove as much threat as possible from a discussion of COPQ. For example, COPQ should not be used as a performance measurement tool for groups or individuals — more harm than good will usually result. It is only when people in one group all feel sure that people in the other group genuinely share their interest in finding the best opportunities for eliminating waste that people will come forward with their special knowledge of how the work really gets done. This is one of the main reasons why TQM/CQI places so much emphasis on building trust.

- It is hard to get people interested in eliminating waste when it may result in eliminating their own job. There is really no honest way to reassure people about this situation. The truth is that an organization has choice only between, on the one hand, actively becoming more effective/competitive and, on the other hand, being passive, which means not surviving at all. In either case, jobs will be lost. To be sure, it is cold comfort to the ones who lose out that this is the price for survival of the organization as a whole. However, experience has shown that people will respect you more, and you will have greater credibility about things you say on other subjects, if you level with them on this admittedly very tough subject. Of course, it is a lot easier to talk about need for greater efficiency when you are in a growth situation. But most healthcare organizations cannot use this argument today because downsizing is going on everywhere.

For these reasons and others, most organizations should be careful about using COPQ as an operations financial control tool in the conventional sense. Successful use for this purpose requires that you have an exceptionally stable operation with sharp definitions of categories of conventional costs, clearly defined lines of responsibility for cost among the various interacting organizational units, and a system for accumulating cost information that is highly reliable, fully accepted, and has a comfortably long track record. We suggest that only healthcare organizations having these characteristics should consider setting up a formal, detailed COPQ reporting and tracking system.

### Do's and Don't's in Using COPQ

- Do keep your eye on the main objective. Don't let terminology details distract your attention.

- Do get participation by all major stakeholders when holding a COPQ estimating session.

- Do try to include people who will not feel personally threatened in COPQ estimating sessions.

- Don't underestimate the effort required to make people comfortable with the estimating process.

- Don't try to disguise the potential headcount implications of waste-elimination activities.

- Don't try to achieve the rigor of a formal accounting system without very careful advance preparation.

# BENCHMARKING THE MOVE TO CAPITATION

Benchmarking and the move to capitation are made for each other. For most institutions making the move to capitation, critically important changes in the financial structure are required, with inadequate previous experience to serve as a reliable guide. The proliferation of seminars, books, and conferences on the subject all attest to the need people have for more insight into how to proceed. It is in just such situations that benchmarking — the process for discovering what is best and how it is achieved — can make its biggest contribution.

There is one apparent drawback, however, to the use of benchmarking for discovering best practices in capitation: the problem of *secrecy*. Capitation is about financial matters and competitive position, the focus of a healthcare organization's business concerns. It is therefore understandable that two institutions that are (or see themselves as being) in competition with each other will not wish to trade information that might lead to competitive advantage for the other party. It is unlikely that such organizations could ever become benchmarking partners.

The problem of secrecy is easily overcome by going further afield. By finding an organization whose catchment geography does not overlap with yours, or whose services are very different from yours, removes most of the barriers to sharing sensitive information. For example, a group health plan serving upper New England and a similar organization serving an area in the Southwest have little to fear from each other. Also, if your needs can be targeted with sufficient precision, it may be possible to go outside healthcare for the information you seek. For example, as we shall discuss later, contract negotiation is at the heart of the changeover to a capitated structure. Any number of businesses in a variety of industrial settings can supply useful insights into the negotiation process.

In order to make the most effective use of benchmarking in capitation, it is necessary to understand the key issues involved. Space does not permit anything like a full exploration of this extremely complex subject in a book of this sort. However, we will discuss one critically important area, namely, *risk management*, in enough detail to provide background for a suggested list of topics related to capitation risk management that are suitable for benchmarking.

## RISK MANAGEMENT

Perhaps more than anything else, capitation is about *financial risk management*. In his book *Against the Gods*, Peter Bernstein defines risk management as follows:

> *The essence of risk management lies in maximizing the areas where we have some control over the outcome while minimizing the areas where we have absolutely no control over the outcome and the linkage between effect and cause is hidden from us (p. 197).*

For healthcare capitation, financial risk management is the estimation, allocation, and reduction of the financial risks associated with contracting to provide a specified set of healthcare services to a defined population at a fixed price per head. We will discuss each of these as it relates to benchmarking, but first it is necessary to understand some things about people's *perceptions of risk* and their *attitudes toward risk*.

Risk is a complicated subject because it is a curious *mélange* of the laws of probability and the laws of human nature. As pointed out in the introductory chapter, one of the purposes of this book is to offer practical advice on how to do benchmarking in the real world of people, where subjective elements such as fear, territoriality, the power imperative, and other emotions all form part of the context for benchmarking. In this real world, nothing is more subjective than our characteristic *personal attitudes toward risk.*

In his book, Peter Bernstein illustrates these attitudes with numerous examples. Here are a few:

- People's *perception* of risk is dominated by qualitative (subjective) rather than quantitative measures. In an experiment people were offered the opportunity to bet on drawing a red ball from an urn that was certified to contain a 50-50, mixture of red and black balls. They were also offered the same wager from another urn with an unknown mixture of red and black balls. Probability theory says that the second urn may as well be considered to be split 50-50, also, because there is no basis for any other distribution, but the overwhelming majority chose to make their bet on the first urn, where the *perceived* uncertainty/risk was less.

- People's *valuation* of something at risk is strongly influenced by whether or not they currently possess it. In one experiment, a group of Cornell students were each given an attractive-looking coffee mug at the beginning of a "seminar." As they were leaving the room at the end of the session, they were offered the opportunity to sell the mug back. The average owner would not sell below $5.25. Another group of Cornell students were shown the same mug at the beginning of a similar session and were told it would be on-sale to them at the end of the session. The average buyer would not pay over $2.25.

  Moreover, this valuation asymmetry (called the "endowment effect" by Richard Thaler, who studied it carefully) appears not to depend too much on whether the thing possessed is desirable or undesirable. In another experiment, a group of people were told to imagine themselves in a situation where there was a one in one thousand chance that they would die suddenly in the morning. They were then asked how much they would pay to have someone else assume that risk. A typical response was about $200.

These same people were then asked how much they would have to be paid to assume this same risk from someone else. A typical reply was a demand for $50,000 as the price of willingness to accept the risk.

- People's "mental accounting" is plagued by *inconsistencies*. Researchers asked subjects to imagine two situations involving theater tickets. In one, the subject discovers, upon arriving at the theater, that he has lost his ticket. Replacement would cost $40. In the other situation, upon arriving at the box office, the subject discovers that he had a hole in his pocket, and has lost $40. The researchers found that most people would not be willing to replace the lost ticket, while about the same number would be willing to buy another ticket even though they had lost an equivalent amount on the way to the theater!

## RISK ESTIMATION: OBJECTIVE AND SUBJECTIVE

As the examples above illustrate, risk is at least as much about human psychology as it is about probability. If it were not for the human side of it, all aspects of risk estimation could be turned over to an actuary. Provided with all the available data, the actuary can identify the risks associated with capitating a given population for a set of defined services. Even with incomplete data (the usual situation, as we all know) the actuary can calculate, for example, the statistical fluctuations to be expected in the incidence of vaginal births after cesarean section (VBAC) for a given population of women of child-bearing age. He can then fold the likelihood of these fluctuations into his calculation of the overall financial risk in a given time period associated with capitating the average cost for normal childbirth for that population. A great many other variables affecting the cost of maternity are also involved, of course, each with its average value and distribution about the average. The calculations can become very tedious, and there is a great deal of uncertainty about the data, but in the hands of a good statistician the process produces a reasonably well-defined objective estimate of risk.

Subjective estimates of risk are another matter entirely. In the obstetrical situation mentioned above, the difficulty lies in gauging the *reaction* of the providers of maternity services when they are asked to accept the risks served up to them by the computer. For example, not all the specialists in providing maternity services will feel comfortable that a dry statistical analysis captures the characteristics of their own practice. How many times have we heard "But our patients are different," often with substantial justification? Nor are all provider panels identical. There will be genuine differences of opinion between panels or even among members of the same panel about, for example, what constitutes best practice for VBAC. Knowledge of such differences will inevitably influence providers' perception of the trustworthiness of the mathematically determined average risk. Couple these concerns about the probabilistically determined risk with the perceptions and attitudes about risk documented by Bernstein and others, and it is readily seen that risk estimates for capitation contracts are not so much tables of data to be published, but issues to be discussed and negotiated with great care and patience by the parties to the negotiation.

> *Risk is at least as much about how people behave in probabilistic situations as it is about probability.*

Benchmarking can provide valuable information about the best way to conduct these negotiations by tapping into the experience of other groups who have wrestled with the same issues. By asking questions and learning about specific approaches to the negotiating process, it is possible to avoid many an awkward impasse.

## RISK ALLOCATION: A SYSTEMS PERSPECTIVE

A **system** is a set of interacting, interdependent parts ("subsystems") aligned to a common purpose. A **systems thinker** is a person who understands the general characteristics of systems, including concepts such as subsystem interactions, feedback loops, etc., and applies them to gain insights into the past and future behavior of a system she/he is studying (P. Senge 1990, 12).

*Risk allocation.* The systems thinker approaches risk in exactly the same way a systems engineer approaches stress allocation — she/he seeks ways to allocate or distribute the stress or the risk across the parts of the system so as to optimize the performance of the system in its operating environment. To understand what this means in practice, let us look at a very simple example.

Consider the system for providing biopsy reports to a surgical team. This system (itself a subsystem of the laboratory system) may be partitioned into a number of parts: for example, transportation, specimen control, specimen preparation, specimen diagnosis, report preparation, and report transmission. A key performance measure for this system is total turnaround time: it should be as short as possible consistent with the other performance criteria.

Imagine that you have been asked to redesign the biopsy process so as to optimize specimen turnaround time. One of the things you must provide is a set of turnaround time requirements to the individual subsystems, dividing up total turnaround time in a rational and equitable way.

Suppose you know all you need to know about how long it has taken historically to carry out each of these subsystem functions, including knowledge of the number of biopsies performed, the distribution of times for each of various categories of specimen, the conditions under which each was processed (time of day, probability of a pile-up of traffic of specimens requiring similar treatment, etc.), and all the other parameters that can influence how long it might take to turn around a given biopsy. You are then in a position to make an equitable *allocation* of the average time to perform each of the functions for each kind of specimen, and to establish ranges of acceptable performance for each.

If the total allowable turnaround time for some category of specimen is one hour, for example, you would not want to allow 15 minutes for transportation and 30 minutes for specimen control, leaving only 15 minutes for all the other process steps. This would be putting undue stress on steps that require more time, and would increase the *risk* that the total turnaround time requirement would not be met. In systems engineering, stress-allocation and risk-allocation are very closely coupled.

Entirely analogous actions would be involved in a purely rational approach to financial risk-allocation under capitation. It will be necessary to make use of all the information available about the population being served, about the providers of the service, about the categories of services to be provided, etc. To be sure, a great deal of probabilistic analysis must be used initially to make up for lack of hard data, but the accumulation of additional experience will enable you to fill in the gaps in your knowledge of how the system actually performs.

This rational approach to risk-allocation has three major advantages over one based on judgment alone:

- It is very likely to produce a fairer and more robust distribution of the financial risk among PCPs, specialists, hospitals, and providers of other services.

- It provides a sound framework for *improving* the allocation as more data become available.

- It provides a departure point that is as quantitative and objective as possible for negotiation among the various parties to a contract to provide capitated services.

- Risk allocation can be determined rationally using proven systems engineering methods.

Next we will discuss the practicalities of trying to *apply* this fully rational approach.

## RISK REDUCTION

We distinguish between *risk reduction* and *risk-shifting*. Risk-shifting is the transfer of risk from one organization to another through, for example, successful negotiating maneuvers. If it results in a disproportionate amount of the risk being borne by one part of the system, risk-shifting does nothing to improve system performance. In the long run it is bound to be destructive.

Under capitation, financial risk is the risk of unpredicted cost, and risk reduction comes down to reduction of unpredictable cost.

Cost of Poor Quality estimates can be an effective tool in capitation to identify functions where the current COPQ is not only high but relatively *unpredictable* — adding to the risk — and to identify where the biggest short-term risk-reduction opportunities are. On a longer time scale, COPQ estimates can also be used to identify where strategic structural changes in the work flow may be desirable in order to make the provider organization able to submit more competitive capitated bids.

However, as we have seen above, there are important barriers to making good COPQ estimates. These barriers are mostly connected with people's behavior, which can be strongly influenced by the capitation model being followed. Whenever two interacting organizations are involved in a COPQ discussion, even when they are two departments in the same hospital, people tend to circle the wagons and prepare to fight. Turf is perceived to be threatened, competence is perceived to be called into question, and denial sets in. A time-consuming process of trust-building is required to overcome these barriers to cooperative effort. Frequent appeals to common interest, reminders that "we are all aligned to achieve the same goals," and similar arguments are all persuasive, but they take time to work.

This tendency to resist attempts to identify the sources of excessive cost will be all the stronger, of course, when the parties to the discussion do not share *any* common organizational allegiance. And when financial risk-allocation is directly tied to people's take-home compensation, progress can be slow indeed. For these reasons, it is desirable to work toward as broad an organizational umbrella as possible for the parties involved in negotiating how they will share the risks associated with a capitated contract.

There are a great many possible models for capitation — at least as many as there are for managed care itself — ranging all the way from hospital-only to full Integrated Care organizations. A typical situation might be one in which a single entity consisting of a hospital plus its staff of PCPs (perhaps organized as an IPA), joins with several other separate groups of specialist providers and ancillary service providers to respond to an RFP from a major employer. Contract negotiations within such a coalition can be very difficult, and no wonder — the coalition is not a system, and the various parties are not aligned with a common (financial) purpose. They *do* have a common purpose when it comes to the desire to provide the best possible care to the subscribers, but this may be of little help when it comes to the administrative and clinical details of how to accomplish this. The financial overlay of who should incur the financial risks associated with the best possible care makes it only that much harder.

Clearly a great many considerations are involved in putting together the right structure for a capitation contract, but *from a purely risk-reduction* perspective, a systems thinker would opt for a global capitation model.

---

### Transition to Capitation Guidelines

- Cost of Poor Quality estimates can be useful in working toward improving your competitive position in a capitated environment.
- Cost and risk allocation negotiations go better when the financial interests of all the providers are aligned.

---

## BENCHMARKING RISK MANAGEMENT IN CAPITATED CONTRACTS

The following questions can be used to establish objectives and goals for benchmarking projects in preparation for the transition to capitated healthcare. They are suitable for use either individually or in various combinations, based on need.

- How do we find out whether the population we plan to serve is appropriate for capitation?
- What is the best way to organize our workforce for capitation. By department? By product line?
- When is the best time to reorganize the workforce — before, during, or after the move to capitated pricing?
- What is the best way to accumulate costs?
- What is the best software package for doing this cost accumulation?
- How do we work effectively with actuaries if we decide to bring them in?
- How should we think about apportioning risk equitably?
- Which is best for us — subcapitation or global? What should we use for criteria? What should we measure?

- If we decide to move into sub-capitation of specialties, is it better to go incrementally or all at once? If incrementally, which specialties are the best to start with?
- How do we go about setting up risk pools?
- How do we deal with people who want to play "risk-shifter"?
- How should contracts be written so that accumulating experience can be used to modify individual portions of the contract without having to start all over again with the negotiations?
- How can we safely develop partnerships with large employers who are capable of helping us into the world of capitated pricing?
- What is the most effective way to work with physicians to identify opportunities for cost reduction while maintaining quality?

### Specific to teaching hospitals and academic medical centers:

- How do we set appropriate cost differentials caused by, for example, different guidelines for utilization review, different severity of illness profiles, different case mixes, etc.?
- How do we negotiate price differentials with buyers?
- How do we deal with increased risk because of adverse selection among providers in an area served by many hospitals? (Other hospitals may effectively follow a risk-shifting strategy, even if only inadvertently.)

# Appendixes

## Appendix 1

# Team Building

*Team* is a much-overworked word. Groups of individuals with widely different backgrounds, skills, and agendas are frequently brought together by well-intentioned management and declared to be "a team." When the members continue to act like individuals with widely different backgrounds, etc., great disappointment results, and "the team approach" is judged to be a fad that won't last. Benchmarking teams are not exempt from this danger. The purpose of this appendix is to offer some guidelines for quickly transforming a collection of individual volunteers into a productive benchmarking team. We will not provide a cookbook recipe, or propose agendas for one or more team-building sessions, but rather address the major barriers that must be overcome to make this transformation.

We define a team as a group of people having diverse skills who are committed to achieving some shared objective.

## SHARED OBJECTIVE

The single biggest act in the formation of a benchmarking team occurs when all the participants together take ownership of the objective. It would be a minor miracle if this were to happen spontaneously. The big cards appear all to be stacked against it:

- The participants were selected *because* they represent different points of view.
- Their prime allegiance is to the department, profession, etc., that is their organizational home.
- They were recruited at least partly for their detailed knowledge of the operation being benchmarked. They will inevitably have beliefs, probably well formulated, about what needs fixing and how to do so.
- They are usually chosen because they are opinion-leaders in their own sphere of influence, and are used to bringing others around to their own point of view, not the reverse.

Against these obstacles, several effective weapons are available. One of these is the protective shield of the power structure. Participants in a benchmarking project must become convinced that in the eyes of executive management the overall objective of the project transcends the interests of any particular affected unit in the organization. (If this were not so, there would be no benchmarking project to begin with.) They must come to believe that a solid set of workable recommendations from the project will be recognized as a valuable contribution to the institution as a whole, and rewarded accordingly.

Another weapon is candor. It should be openly acknowledged that participants in a benchmarking project are both members of a team *and* representatives from their home organization. They will both be expected to show team solidarity *and* be expected to bring the viewpoints of those they represent to the study and argue for their interests. Being a representative in two directions at once is not easy. When participants feel that the difficulty of their assignment is understood and appreciated by management, the situation becomes more tolerable.

The job of the person leading the team-building session(s) is to maintain an atmosphere in which the participants can work their way through the issues together. A few pointers are:

- Don't hesitate to start with an ice-breaker. The cornier the better, some say, as long as it is clever and fresh. People all like to have fun.
- Early in the session, state the overall objective of the project and ask for each participant's reactions. (It is helpful if the team spon-

sor leads this part of the discussion.) Then state the proposed benchmarking project goal, emphasizing that one of the team's first jobs will be to sharpen and refine this goal statement.

- Go around the table at frequent intervals. Every time an important new point comes up, give each participant two to three minutes to speak to it freely. The exchange of views usually reveals that most of the issues and anxieties are seen in about the same way by everyone.

- Leave plenty of time for unstructured venting. After a time, people begin to realize that most of the concerns have been dealt with before.

- Do not try to respond point by point to every concern as it is expressed. Wait until points have been made more than once, then either give the facts or promise to get the facts if you don't have them.

- Don't try to do this part of team building all in one session. People need time to reflect, seek peer opinion, and come to terms with what they have learned. Be prepared for a rehash of some aspect or other of the original discussion at any time during the first few team meetings.

See Action planning for a discussion of the team-building aspects of planning and implementing the action recommendations.

## DIVERSE SKILLS

A benchmarking team *needs* diverse skills: healthcare work is complicated, and no one knows how to do it all. But along with the diversity in skills come diversities in style, language, and experience that can erect formidable barriers to communication and smooth working relationships. To overcome these barriers a team needs procedures for working together that everyone understands and agrees with. A major part of team building is to help the group develop these procedures, which include *rules* about such activities as:

- *Preparing input.* Most groups soon discover that meeting time is precious, and that some kinds of communication cannot be hurried.

249

They learn to do as much of the work as possible outside the meetings. This permits people to work in parallel on different parts of the same analysis, document, etc. When the team members agree to this pattern at the very beginning, much valuable time is saved.

- *Debating.* One of the great strengths of a group effort is that it enables different viewpoints to rub up against each other, and this guarantees disagreements. Properly disciplined, the ensuing debates lead to much illumination but not too much heat. The group needs to assess candidly its own behavioral profile — i.e., what kind of a mix of personality types are represented on the team — and decide on appropriate ground rules for debates. These can be quite formal at first (e.g., requiring someone who is about to disagree with a statement to restate it before plunging in), loosening up as people get to know each other and group behavioral norms become established.

- *Decision-making.* The decision-making process is a continuum, ranging all the way from pure dictatorship to unanimous acclamation. A consensus (everyone can say "My views have been heard and fairly considered. I may not agree with the majority position in all details, but I will support the decision wholeheartedly") is usually considered optimal.

  Various voting procedures (nominal group technique, paired comparisons, etc.) are ordinarily used to discover how the group is leaning, as a guide to where a discussion should be concentrated. It is a good idea to use one of these procedures — the simpler the better — as a time saver to avoid needless discussion of some option that no one, not even the person who proposed it, takes very seriously.

  At the end of the project there will be important decisions to be made about the recommendations and their wording. It is well to establish a pattern of orderly decision-making well in advance of these deliberations so that you can honestly say the actions that you propose are a real team consensus. Practice makes perfect.

- *Documentation.* Group activities produce all manner of meeting notes, flip-charts, homework handouts, etc. Rules for how these should be produced and saved need to be developed. A good

250

general rule is: keep it simple. For example, the meeting minutes should not attempt to be a substitute for attendance at the meetings. Restricting the minutes to include only decisions and action item assignments may be somewhat too Spartan, but is at the right end of the spectrum.

See Meeting Ground Rules and Meeting Roles in the Blood Bank case study for examples of the output from a team-building session.

## ACHIEVING THE OBJECTIVE

Most groups bring plenty of knowledge to a benchmarking project. But there are barriers to getting it out of the individual heads and accepted into the team's working knowledge, where it can contribute to achieving the project objective. Overcoming these barriers requires the use of group process tools, of which the most useful are those which help the communication process — bringing in and transferring information, organizing it, and fitting it into place.

If the team participants are already familiar with these tools, a quick refresher at the team building session may be appropriate. If not, training is indicated.

We are firm proponents of just-in-time training, and believe that training at team-building sessions should be targeted at the tools that the team can use *immediately* to get the project moving. These might include such topics as brainstorming, affinity diagrams with Post-it notes, tree diagrams, and other nonesoteric data organizing tools such as Pareto charts, bar graphs, and histograms.

One tool, *work process flow-charting*, is so important in benchmarking that it needs special consideration. Because flow-charting is profoundly *a group tool* — nobody knows it all — it is valuable to have the team learn and practice it together. If some members of the team are already familiar with flow-charting and others are not, one approach to this training is to use it as an ice-breaker. Dividing the team into two subgroups, you might try Getting Ready for a Family Vacation or a Neighborhood Barbecue or something fun like that. Those with experience can help the neophytes. Mention that flow-charting software is available for use when the team gets to Step 3.

251

# Appendix 2

# Preparing Questionnaires

The questionnaire is one of the most valuable tools in benchmarking, but one of the hardest to master. If at all possible, people who are inexperienced in questionnaire construction should *always* take advantage of others who have some experience. In Chapter 1 we discussed the *content* of the questions. In this Appendix we will talk about the *structure* of the questions and the *process* for team development of the questionnaire.

## STRUCTURE: WORDING

The wording of a question is critically important. (Recall the ancient joke about the man who didn't know what to say when asked "Have you stopped beating your wife?") When reviewing your questions for effective wording, put yourself in the position of the person who is trying to answer them.

Questions come in many forms:

1. *Forced-choice.* The most unambiguous. Example: Does your pharmacy use the same patient-numbering system as the pathology lab? (Yes or no.) Usually followed up with a question leading into more detail.

2. *Multiple-choice.* Allows for more detail. For example, the follow-up question to the pharmacy question above might be: If so, who is responsible for ensuring that the numbers actually are the same? (Admitting, Medical Records, Pharmacy. Lab, Other.) Note the

use of the category called "Other." This category is needed when you are not sure if you have all the possibilities covered, which may be frequently.

3. *Scaled.* Watch out for these. If your scale is in terms of a range of numbers (e.g., 0 – 25; 25 – 75; 75 – 100), all well and good. But if it is in terms of judgments (e.g., Not important; Somewhat important; Very important), you have a calibration problem that can make data interpretation difficult.

4. *Open-ended questions.* Watch out for these, too. The responses can't be tabulated, the responses may be too brief to be useful, or they may be too long and have to be summarized. Moreover, they suggest that you have not thought carefully about what you want to learn, and respondents will generally hate them. Horrible example: In fifty words or less, how do you avoid return to the OR from the ICU?

To illustrate the importance of *how a question is structured*, consider the following example (Bernstein 1996, 278) of what can happen to the answers to a multiple-choice question depending on the choices offered. Two groups of physicians were presented with an incomplete case history and a list of possible diagnoses. The first group was presented with a list having two possible specific diagnoses, A and B, and a third option, "none of the above." The second group was presented with a list having *five* possible specific diagnoses, A, B, C, D, and E, plus the "none of the above" option. Here are the results:

| Group 1 | | Group 2 | |
|---|---|---|---|
| possible diagnosis | probability | possible diagnosis | probability |
| A<br>B } | 50% | A<br>B<br>C } | 31% |
| none of the above } | 50% | D<br>E<br>none of the above } | 69% |

The oddity, of course, is that two diagnoses, A and B, which were given a combined probability of 50% by the first group of physicians, were given only a 31% probability by the second group of physicians, simply because the second group was provided with three additional specific possible diagnoses.

# STRUCTURE: FORMATTING

Be sure that the overall organization of the questionnaire is *user-friendly*. The different sections should be clearly marked. There should be enough space for the reply, even if the answer requires only a few words. Multiple-choice questions should be arranged similarly on the page — the respondent should not have to play hide-and-seek looking for answer boxes in a variety of locations.

# PROCESS

When developing a questionnaire, all members of the team should be encouraged to submit possible questions. If this is their first experience, it is best not to worry about categorizing the questions at first submission.

After the initial submission, **screener-type** questions (questions that will be most useful in determining the suitability of a contact as a benchmarking partner) should be segregated into a **screener list**. This list, suitably augmented with important questions based on information obtained from library-type inquiries, should then be converted into a **screener questionnaire**. (See Figure 9 in of the Blood Bank case for an example of a screener questionnaire.)

The remaining questions, perhaps 50–100, need to be organized into a second questionnaire, the detailed one. One very effective organization is according to who will answer the questionnaire in the partnering organization. For example, questions to be answered by the nursing staff should be arranged together, those for pharmaceuticals, ditto, etc. This will be useful irrespective of whether the benchmarking partner institution is organized into traditional departments or by product line, because the emphasis is on learning how the work is done.

An easy way to organize the questionnaire is to assign one member of the benchmarking team for each type of respondent (nursing, pharmaceutical, etc.) and have them develop their own section of the questionnaire outside the team meeting. This can be a good check on team composition — if these assignments do not come naturally, the team's mix of professional specialties may need adjustment. This work can and should be done in parallel to save time. Don't worry yet that some questions will appear in more than one section of the questionnaire. Some overlap will turn out to be appropriate.

After the organizing work is done, the team should review the draft questionnaire. A full team meeting can be profitably devoted to this activity. A few tips for carrying out the review:

- Ask yourself if you really need the answer to this question.

- Check to be sure that you cannot answer the question yourself with library-type data.

- Ask yourself if the question is completely unambiguous:
  - Could the respondent misinterpret the question?
  - Could you misinterpret the answer?

- Organize the questions to have a natural order: by topic, and usually from the more general to the more specific.

- Check to be sure that redundant use of a question in different sections is appropriate.

- Always put yourself in the position of the person answering the question.

# Appendix 3
# Action Planning

This appendix is about how you as a member of the benchmarking team can help with action planning in Phase IV. Your assignment is to provide support to the group of people — from here on "the group" for short — who will be accountable for the detailed planning and for carrying out the action plan recommended by the benchmarking team. It is assumed that you have been designated by the team for this role either because you are a member of "the group" or have other special skills and abilities that make you a logical choice for this role.

You will be building on the experience you have already gained in Phase I while planning the benchmarking project itself. Recall that Step 1 in Phase I culminates in a document called the **team charter**, which comprises:

- Project scope and constraints
- Measures of success
- Resources
- Output
- Team schedule

This team charter is, in fact, the benchmarking project plan. It describes *what* will be done, *who* will do it, *why* it will be done, *how* it will be done, in what *sequence*, and according to what *schedule* the actions will occur.

Recall also that you arrived at this plan or charter in a series of discussions in which you:

- Came to a full understanding of the objective, why its achievement is important to the organization, and aligned a collection of individuals into a team committed to making it happen.

257

- Agreed on the scope and detailed wording of the objective.
- Reached understanding of what must be done to accomplish the objective, and developed measures of success.
- Translated these needs into assignments, resource requirements, and a schedule of activities.
- Tested the sturdiness of the parts of the plan and how they fit together.

Remember how it felt to go through this sequence of events? It was a necessary part of the human dynamics of planning the benchmarking project. The Japanese call this sequence "nemawashi" — literally "root-binding" — what a gardener does in preparation for transplanting a tree or bush to a new location in the garden. In the context of the benchmarking project, the *nemawashi* process was required in order to prepare the benchmarking team to transplant new or improved processes from the outside world into your own organization.

Now the *nemawashi* process must be repeated in order to prepare *the group* for its task of transplanting the new or improved process into its permanent home in the organization, and under their ongoing care. A benchmarking team member — one who has gone through all of this before — is in a strong position to help make this step a success, particularly if that benchmarking team member is also a trusted and respected member of the group.

If you are not yourself already a member of the group, offer to serve as a **facilitator** — someone who helps to make meetings a success. A good facilitator has knowledge of both the subject matter and good meeting dynamics, but uses her/his subject matter knowledge only sparingly, and mostly to enable good meeting dynamics. (Remember — one of your goals is to transfer process ownership to the group.) If the group for whatever reason does not take you up on your offer to facilitate, do not back off completely, but continue to hold yourself in readiness to supply information, perspective, and enthusiasm.

If you *are* a member of the group and served as its representative on the benchmarking team, perhaps even as team leader, there is still a lot to be said for offering to be the facilitator during the early stages of planning.

The sequence of activities in Phase IV: Action Planning should go something like the following:

1. The first thing the group has to do is understand and accept the objective driving the recommended actions. This is no small task. Expect that there will be all sorts of questions, objections, and expressions of skepticism about the wisdom/doability/desirability. Arrange for a person in higher management to kick off the first meeting of the planning group, emphasizing the importance of the work and the management commitment to its success. It is a good investment, in any case, but can make the difference between success and failure when the objective is to bring in a *new* process where it is very likely that a freshly formed collection of individuals has been assembled to make it happen.

   The role of the process owner/group manager at this meeting is to answer the questions and lead the discussion. The main job of the facilitator is to prepare the process owner to do so. If the facilitator is a benchmarking team member or the team leader, do not become defensive and leap in with detailed explanations during this meeting. Leave plenty of time for people to come to terms with the detailed substance of something that they know only in broad outline so far.

2. The group should next study the process flow chart. If the action recommendations are for improvements to the existing process, the group is already familiar with its flow chart, having participated in producing it for the benchmarking team in Step 3 of Phase I. The discussion can focus immediately on understanding the content of the proposed modifications.

   If the action is to introduce a new process, for example, the introduction of a new treatment for ischemic stroke, as in the second case study, more time will be needed for the group to become familiar with the accompanying flowchart. Here the facilitator should distribute copies of the flow chart to everyone affected prior to the meeting, and again prepare the group leader to answer questions and lead the discussion. Also, the requirements of the team-building process must be factored in, but a properly handled discussion of the process flow chart is an excellent team-building vehicle, and need not be deferred on that account.

3. To help the group get started thinking about what needs to be done, suggest that they begin by constructing an **affinity diagram** of all their ideas. When this is done, it oftentimes looks like a simple modified tree diagram with the objective at the top and key elements of the objective serving as category headings for lists of people, methods, and things that may have to be considered. For example, in the roll-out planning for the new stroke protocol in the second case, such a diagram might have looked like this:

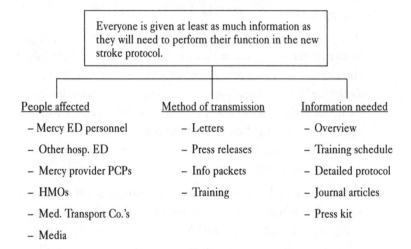

Everyone is given at least as much information as they will need to perform their function in the new stroke protocol.

| People affected | Method of transmission | Information needed |
| --- | --- | --- |
| – Mercy ED personnel | – Letters | – Overview |
| – Other hosp. ED | – Press releases | – Training schedule |
| – Mercy provider PCPs | – Info packets | – Detailed protocol |
| – HMOs | – Training | – Journal articles |
| – Med. Transport Co.'s | | – Press kit |
| – Media | | |

Another approach is to construct a conventional tree diagram directly, with the objective on the left, and progressively more detailed categories of activity (answers to the question "How?") as the tree fans out to the right. You can check the *need* for the branches of the tree by moving back to the left on the tree, to progressively more general categories of activity, asking the question "Why?" about each branch as you go.

4. Next comes the nitty-gritty of deciding how much effort and how much time will be required to put the new improved process into routine operation. Quite commonly people will say, "How can I know how much effort it will take to do this task?" Very

often the best answer is that you can't. But an estimate can be made, and the parts of the estimate (perhaps broken out to coincide with specific boxes on the tree diagram) are individually capable of surprisingly accurate projections. Eat the 500-pound marshmallow one bite at a time.

Or they may say, "How can I know how long it will take to do this task?" Again the best answer may be that you can't. But you can still establish a target date and develop a rough draft set-back schedule, which you can revise as you get deeper into the details of the plan.

Sometimes a deadline for full implementation of the new or improved process is imposed from outside by management, and the group discovers that it can't meet the deadline. In such a case, a carefully prepared set-back schedule, or Gantt chart, becomes very useful in negotiating a more realistic deadline.

5. The group is now ready to ask themselves what *measurements* they would want to make at major mileposts to show progress toward the objective. Many of these measurements will turn out to be very similar to, or the same as, the ones that the benchmarking team used to establish the gap between your organization's performance and that of the benchmark. New measurements not part of the present data gathering system may be proposed. Measurements that relate to time, cost, and critical performance parameters are all potentially OK, but it is better to have a *few* of the *right* measures than many unimportant measures that only tend to obscure the situation.

6. When all the major elements of the plan — the what, the who, the how much, the how long, and the major mileposts, have been roughed out by the group as a whole, it is time for a few people to put it all together. Be sure to get the financial people involved at this stage. The operational consequence of successful benchmarking is that the operating plan changes, and that's their baby. Moreover, they have software to produce helpful progress-tracking tools such as Gantt charts and even PERT charts, in cases where the plan is sufficiently complex to require their use.

7. Distribute copies of the completed plan for study by all members of the group prior to a meeting to review and commit to the plan and assume ownership of it.

Finally, keep in mind that there will be resistance to the very idea of making an implementation plan. Many of us avoid planning when at all possible. We tell ourselves that we don't need a plan; we know pretty much what to do. Or we say that we won't need a plan; we can figure out what to do next as we go along. However, any action that involves important changes in the way things get done requires management concurrence, and nothing is going to happen in a well-run institution if we just say "trust me." So we have to produce a plan. Don't worry if the crystal ball is cloudy at the beginning; getting started focuses the thinking, and you can always revise the plan.

# Related Resources

## Benchmarking

Camp, R. C. (1989). *Benchmarking*. New York: Quality Resources; and Milwaukee: ASQC Quality Press.

Gift, R. G., and D. Mosel (1994). *Benchmarking in Healthcare: A Collaborative Approach*. Chicago: American Hospital Publishing, Inc.

Watson, G. H. (1993). *Strategic Benchmarking*. New York: John Wiley and Sons.

Watson, G. H. (1992). *The Benchmarking Workbook*. Cambridge, MA: Productivity Press.

## TQM/CQI

Brassard, M. (1989). *The Memory Jogger Plus*. Methuen, NY: Goal-QPC.

Deming, W. E. (1982). *Out of the Crisis*. Cambridge, MA: MIT-CAES.

Juran, J. M. (1988). *Juran s Quality Control Handbook*. 4th ed. New York: McGraw-Hill.

## TQM/CQI in Healthcare

Ayres, I., and J. Braithwaite (1992). *Responsive Regulation: Transcending the Deregulation Debate*. New York: Oxford University Press.

Berwick, D. M., A. B. Godfrey, and J. Roessner, J. (1990). *Curing Health Care*. San Francisco: Jossey-Bass.

Brennan, T. A., and D. M. Berwick (1996). *New Rules*. San Francisco: Jossey-Bass.

Caldwell, C. (1995). *Mentoring Strategic Change in Health Care*. Milwaukee: ASQC Quality Press.

Griffith, J. R., V. K. Sahney, and R. A. Mohr (1995). *Reengineering Health Care*. Ann Arbor: Health Administration Press.

Schifman, R. B., P. J. Horowitz, and R. J. Zarbo (1996). *Advances in Pathology*. Vol. 9: 83–120.

## Internet

Aleks, N. (1997). *Mailing List Management Software FAQ*. Send an e-mail message to: ListProc@avs.com containing the line "get doc mlm software-faq."

Bloom, F. E. (1996). "An Internet Review: the Complete Neuroscientist Scours the World Wide Web." *Science*. Vol. 274: 1104–1108.

Brenner, A. E. (October 1996). "The Computing Revolution and the Physics Community." *Physics Today:* 24–30.

Fukuyama, F. (December 2, 1996). "Trust Still Counts in a Virtual World." *Forbes ASAP*: 33.

Kovacs, D. and M. Strangelove (1991). *Directory of Electronic Journals, Newsletters, and Academic Discussion Lists*. Washington, DC: Association of Research Libraries, Office of Scientific and Academic Publishing. Updated semiannually.

Schatz, B. R. (1997). "Information Retrieval in Digital Libraries: Bringing Search to the Net." *Science*. Vol. 275: 327–334.

The Electronic Frontier Foundation. "EFF s Guide to the Internet: v.2.3." http://www.eff.org/papers/bdgtti/eegtti.html.

Van Alstyne, M. and E. Brynjolfsson (1996). "Could the Internet Balkanize Science?" *Science*. Vol. 274: 1479–1480.

"Special Report on Internet Communities." (May 5, 1997). *Business Week:* 65.

"The Internet: Fulfilling the Promise." (March 1997). *Scientific American:* 68–83.

# Index

# Index

of views to concerned parties, 47-48
Communication process, 58-61
    administrative staff in, 60
    executive committee in, 60-61
    process owner in, 59-60
    workforce in, 60
Conferences, national, 20
Conferencing programs, 215
Confidentiality, 75
Conformance, cost of, 232, 233
Consensus building, 2, 63-64
Consortium Benchmarking Studies, 22
Constraints, 16
Consultants
    consulting firms, 22
    internal consultants/advisors, 15
Content, of communication process, 61-64
    findings, 61, 62
    recommendations, 61, 62-64
Continuous Quality Improvement (CQI),
    4, 5, 23, 84-85, 97, 234
Corporate strategy, 10
Cost of poor quality (COPQ), 231-235
    cost of conformance and, 232, 233
    cost of nonconformance and, 232-233
    do's and don't's of using, 235
    risk reduction and, 242
    traps in using, 233-235
Cost(s)
    allocation of, 226-228
    benchmarking healthcare, 225-245
    control and reduction of, 18, 230-231
    cost of poor quality (COPQ), 231-235,
        242
    definition of, 226, 228
    of Internet benchmarking, 218
    justification of, for new initiatives, 164-
        165
    measurement of, 228-231
    and move to capitation, 236-245
Cranbrook HMO modernization crisis
    (case), 80, 167-187
    action phase, 183-187
    case setting, 167-169
    planning phase, 174-182

project leader, 181-187
Customer
    defined, 5
    sponsor as immediate, 6, 7

Data analysis, 3, 40-44
    compiling responses, 40-41
    identifying benchmarks, 41-42
    identifying gap profile, 42-43
    Internet resources and, 221-222
    pitfalls of, 52
    reviewing findings, 43-44
Data collection and analysis phase, 37-52,
    69
    for Blood Bank at Good Samaritan
        Hospital (case), 111-120
    checklist for, 51
    data analysis, 3, 40-44, 52, 221-222
    identifying best practices, 3, 38, 44-48,
        52, 222
    Internet resources and, 221-222
    overview of, 3
    pitfalls of, 36, 52
    preparation for. *See* Preparing to collect
        data
    questionnaire administration, 3, 38-40,
        52, 221
    site visits, 3, 48-51, 52, 222
Deadlines, for questionnaire completion,
    39
Direct costs, 227
Discussion groups, Internet, 210-213
Doctorow, E. L., 72
Document sharing "white boards," 213-
    214

Electronic mail (e-mail), 208-209
    administering questionnaires through,
        39, 41, 221
    in benchmarking of project, 220
    chat rooms and, 213, 215
    discussion groups via, 210-213
    document sharing "white boards," 213-
        214
    threading, 212, 215

267

# Index

# Index

# Index

*Also available from Quality Resources...*

**The Basics of Benchmarking**
*Robert Damelio*
80 pp., 1995, Item No. 763012, paperback

**The Basics of Process Mapping**
*Robert Damelio*
77 pp., 1996, Item No. 763160, paperback

**Healthcare Redesign Tools and Techniques**
*Jean Ann Larson*
192 pp., 1997, Item No. 763225, hardcover

**Measuring Quality Improvement in Healthcare: A Guide to Statistical Process Control Applications**
*Raymond G. Carey, Ph.D., and Robert C. Lloyd, Ph.D.*
214 pp., 1995, Item No. 762938, paperback

**Strategic Planning in Healthcare: Building a Quality-Based Plan Step by Step**
*Bernard J. Horak, Ph.D., FACHE*
224 pp., 1997, Item No. 763144, hardcover

**Quality Assessment for Healthcare: A Baldrige-Based Handbook**
*Ned Barber, Ph.D.*
204 pp., 1996, Item No. 763055, paperback

**Value-Based Cost Management for Healthcare: Linking Costs to Quality and Delivery**
*Kicab Castañeda-Méndez*
189 pp., 1996, Item No. 763047, hardcover

**Benchmarking: The Search for Industry Best Practices That Lead to Superior Performance**
*Robert C. Camp*
299 pp., 1989, Item No. 916358, hardcover

**For additional information on any of the above titles or for our complete catalog, call 800-247-8519 or 212-979-8600.**

**Visit us at www.qualityresources.com**
**E-mail: info@qualityresources.com**

**Quality Resources, 902 Broadway, New York, NY 10010**